YOUR PERSONAL H

ENDORSE

THE CANADIAN MEDICAL ASSOCIATION

Eyes

Marvin L. Kwitko, MD
and
Marvin Ross

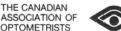 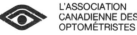

THE CANADIAN
ASSOCIATION OF
OPTOMETRISTS

L'ASSOCIATION
CANADIENNE DES
OPTOMÉTRISTES

KEY PORTER·BOOKS

This book is dedicated to
Lara Ursula Kwitko and Adam Bradley Kwitko

The publisher gratefully acknowledges the assistance of the Canada Council, the Ontario Arts Council and the Ontario Publishing Centre.

Canadian Cataloguing in Publication Data

Kwitko, Marvin L.
  Eyes

(Your personal health series)
Includes index.
ISBN 1-55013-529-5

1. Eye – Diseases and defects – Popular works.
2. Eye – Care and hygiene – Popular works. I. Title.
II. Series.

RE51.K9 1994   617.7   C94-931453-6

Key Porter Books Limited
70 The Esplanade
Toronto, Ontario
Canada M5E 1R2

Design: Maher Design
Diagrams: Martyn Lengden
Typesetting: MACTRIX DTP
Printed and bound in Canada

94 95 96 97 98 6 5 4 3 2 1

Contents

INTRODUCTION

The eye is a fascinating organ. It works on simple principles of light refraction, yet it performs with extraordinary accuracy and flexibility. It is in many ways a delicate instrument, yet it has a remarkable ability to adapt or recuperate. Man's search for solutions to the problems of vision has been an incredible journey in intellectual discovery. People have been trying to understand and solve vision problems since the days of ancient Babylon, and before. We are fortunate that, in our own era, medical science has made great strides in correcting eye problems. We also have the benefit of many ingenious devices and techniques to help people with poor vision, or no vision, lead productive lives. In the years to come, perhaps we will finally learn to cure blindness and, even if we can't restore sight, to dramatically improve the lives of the blind.

The first chapter of this book explains the basic principles of how the eye works, and introduces the vocabulary of the eye. Unless you read this fundamental information, you may find the rest of the book hard to understand. Later chapters deal with specific areas of eye problems, so that readers can focus on their own particular concerns. We hope everyone will read Chapter Seven, a brief guide to eye emergencies; a few minutes invested here may prevent serious damage.

Although medical terms are explained as they appear, you will find a handy glossary of these terms at the end of the book. There is also a comprehensive index.

O N E

The Anatomy of the Eye

To the poet, the eye is the window of the soul; to the physician, it is a window on the state of our health. To most of us, it provides close to 80 percent of the information we need to evaluate the environment around us. All this in a structure that weighs a mere 7 g and is only about 2.5 cm in diameter.

Because eyes are so important, nature has provided safety devices to protect them from injury. The eyes are set back in the eye sockets, or orbits, in a bony mass so they are shielded by the cheekbones, the bridge of the nose, and the brow. The eyelids close reflexively to protect against dust and objects thrust towards the eye. ("Reflexively" means that we don't have to think about blinking to protect our eyes; we do it automatically.) Tear glands are located in the outer corners of

The Human Eye

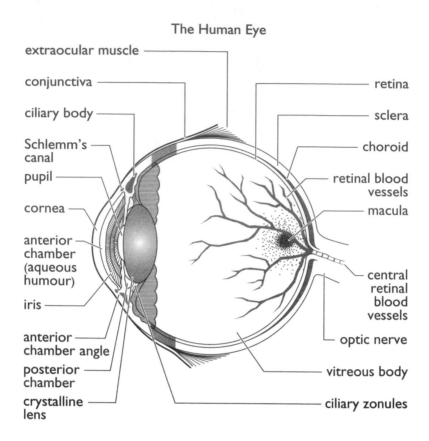

extraocular muscle

conjunctiva

ciliary body

Schlemm's canal

pupil

cornea

anterior chamber (aqueous humour)

iris

anterior chamber angle

posterior chamber

crystalline lens

retina

sclera

choroid

retinal blood vessels

macula

central retinal blood vessels

optic nerve

vitreous body

ciliary zonules

the upper lids, and continually moisten the eye to keep it clean and free of tiny particles. Finally, for further protection, most parts of the eye are hidden away. The only parts exposed are the sclera, covered by conjunctiva and the cornea.

The *sclera* is the white, outer part of the eye. It's a tough, protective coat of collagen and elastic tissue. The *pupil* is the hole (or aperture) through which light passes into the eye. The size of the pupil changes depending upon the amount of light present; the greater the amount of light, the smaller the pupil.

The Telltale Pupil

Eckhard H. Hess, a psychologist at the University of Chicago, has carried out research projects that indicate that the pupil may very well be a "window to our soul." In one study, men and women were presented with male and female "stimulus pictures" and the size of their pupils was photographed and measured. The men's pupils dilated more when presented with a female pinup picture. Women's pupils dilated more when shown pictures of babies, a mother and a baby, and a male pinup.

In another study, men were shown identical pictures of women, but half the women had their pictures retouched with smaller pupils and half with larger pupils. The men responded more favourably to the pictures with the larger pupils, even though they stated that the pictures were identical. Large pupils, it seems, are attractive to men. But then, this isn't news. In the past, some women deliberately dilated their pupils with belladonna (a dangerous poison also called atropine); the name means "beautiful woman."

In the final study, a group of men were given arithmetic problems and their pupil size was measured before and after each problem. The more difficult the problem, the greater the increase in pupil size — but men who were skilled in arithmetic had a smaller increase in pupil size. The pupil, Hess concluded, is a sensitive measure of a variety of activities going on in the brain.

This is why it takes us a few seconds to adjust to a change in light. When we first go out into bright sunshine, we must squint until the pupil constricts and limits the amount of light getting through. When we enter a dark room, we see little or nothing until the pupil expands to let more light in.

The *iris* is the coloured area surrounding the pupil. It contains two major sets of muscles that dilate and constrict (open and close) the pupil. It also contains numerous blood vessels and pigment cells; the pigment cells give the iris its different colours of blue, green, hazel, and brown.

The *conjunctiva* is a filmy, transparent membrane that covers and protects the sclera and lines the inner side of the eyelids. It too contains many blood vessels, which may

---

Taking care of your eyes

Although many conditions affecting the front portion of the eye can be corrected, damage to the back areas — such as the retina, choroid, and optic nerve — is often permanent. Much of the harm done to these sensitive areas could easily be prevented.

Sunglasses are an essential protection against glare and dangerous ultraviolet rays. They are especially important when you are around water or snow, because you may be exposed to more glare than you realize, due to reflection. It's not enough to choose dark-coloured lenses; read the labels, and pick a pair of glasses that screen out 60 percent of UVA (longer-wave ultraviolet) and 95 percent of UVB (short-wave ultraviolet). For sunning and skiing, look for even higher ratings.

Never look directly at the sun, even with the strongest sunglasses. Although you may feel no discomfort at the time, the result can be permanent damage or even blindness. Too many people have lost their vision forever because they thought they could watch an eclipse "just for a minute or two."

Always use the appropriate eye protection for work or hobbies, whether it be sport goggles, a helmet visor, or safety glasses for do-it-yourself projects. Develop the habit of keeping your hands away from your eyes, and teach children to do the same. Many substances that your hands can tolerate (such as gritty materials, bacteria, mild cleaning agents, or cooking spices) can create serious problems if they are absent-mindedly rubbed in your eyes.

---

rupture spontaneously, resulting in a very red eye. This clears up without treatment in several days. Your doctor will call this a subconjunctival haemorrhage.

The *cornea* is a clear, transparent membrane that covers the iris and pupil but is separated from them. It is crucial for proper vision. It is about 12 mm in diameter, and thicker at the edges than in the middle. (In the middle it's about 0.5 mm thick, whereas it's about 1 mm thick at the edges.)

The cornea consists of five layers of tissue, and contains numerous small nerve fibres but no blood vessels. It is the first part of the eye through which light passes. The light rays are bent (refracted) so they pass through the pupil and the crystalline lens (see below) and are focused at the back of the eye, on the retina. Good vision requires a crystal-clear cornea. The five layers of the cornea function exclusively to balance the fluid content of the cornea, so that it retains this clarity throughout life.

Disturbances in the curvature of the cornea result in nearsightedness, farsightedness, and astigmatism. Glasses and contact lenses, or surgery of the cornea, can correct these visual problems. In addition, if the cornea loses its clarity through injury or disease, a corneal transplant can be performed; this is the most frequent form of organ transplant done today.

The *crystalline lens* is behind the iris and pupil. Its shape can be changed by muscles in the area called the ciliary body, to focus the rays of light onto the back of the eye (the retina), depending on our distance from the object we're looking at. As we get older, changes in the lens can result in the formation of cataracts, cloudy areas in the lens that cause blurred, hazy vision. Cataracts may affect our distance vision (for driving, for example), or our near vision (for reading), depending on their location.

The area in front of the lens, the *anterior chamber*, is divided into two parts by the iris. Both contain a watery solution called the *aqueous humour*. The angle of the anterior chamber is bounded by the cornea and the iris, and contains part of the ciliary body called the *trabeculum* and the aqueous drainage channel called *Schlemm's canal*. Blockage of the aqueous drainage channel can cause a sudden rise in internal eye pressure when the peripheral iris root blocks Schlemm's canal—a condition called acute glaucoma—or a slow, chronic rise in pressure called open-angle glaucoma, when sclerosis of the trabeculum occurs because of ageing or genetic makeup.

The Sacred Eye

In ancient Egypt, the eye was the symbol of the sun god Ra, who had all-seeing power. Embalmed bodies were given amulets bearing the eye of Osiris, god of the underworld, to guide the soul through the afterlife. Eyes were also painted on mummy shrouds. The protective eye of Horus, the falcon-headed sky god, was often worn as a talisman and even painted on the prow of ships.

Ancient Japanese and Polynesian religions also associated the eye with the sun, which was often considered to represent the eye of the god and creator. In Greek mythology, the eye was the symbol of strength, clarity, and power. The eye has also appeared as symbolism in various South Sea cultures, and among some North American indigenous tribes.

The cavity behind the lens is filled with a jelly-like substance called the *vitreous body*. The aqueous humour and the vitreous body help the lens focus incoming light.

The lens is suspended in place by the *ciliary zonules*, which extend from the *ciliary body*. When the ciliary muscles contract, the elastic lens changes shape to focus the rays of light on the retina. This is called accommodation, because the lens accommodates vision at varying distances.

The *choroid* is a dark brown layer between the sclera and the retina. It consists of blood vessels joined by connective tissue containing pigmented cells, and its main role is to provide nourishment to the retina.

At the back of the eye is the *retina*. This is the nerve-cell layer, and it acts like the film in a camera. It is a thin, transparent tissue containing 120 million rod-shaped cells and 7 million cone-shaped cells. The *macula* is the sensitive central part of the retina, and it provides sharp, detailed vision.

At the very centre of the macula is the *fovea*, which has the highest percentage of cone cells of any area in the macula.

The Evil Eye

Ancient Babylonians thought the eye was governed by a particularly malevolent demon, and any demon or evil spirit that took charge of a body could attack others through the eyes.

The Greeks even feared the reflection of their own eyes. When Damoetas saw himself in a transparent pool, he spat three times at his image to ward off his own evil eye. Plutarch believed the eye threw off both good and bad rays, while Helidorus claimed that anyone looking at someone with envy transmitted a poison that infected the other person's eyes.

The Romans expanded the mythology. Plinius said that certain women of South Russia could kill men and wither plants with one look, and noted that laws were passed to prevent people from destroying crops this way. By the Middle Ages, the evil eye was held responsible for epidemics and sick cattle as well as ruined crops. The bubonic plague was believed to be spread by glances.

Children and pregnant women were considered most vulnerable to the evil eye. Protection was found in the wearing of amulets or in words and gestures. A "horn" made with the index and baby fingers and pointed at the suspected owner of the evil eye was a common protection.

Because of the presence of so many cone cells, the fovea is crucial for defining objects clearly — for reading, for example. Without the fovea, you would not see clearly.

How we see

When rays of light converge on the retina, they stimulate the rod and cone cells. The rods enable us to see in low levels of illumination (for night vision) and do not reach maximum effectiveness for about five minutes (this is called "dark adaptation" and is a second reason why we need time to adapt our vision to darkness). The cones enable us to see in bright illumination, to see details and colour. The cone cells contain pigments that are responsible for colour vision.

As we get older, problems in the retina can affect our vision unless treated quickly. Conditions such as detached retina, diabetic retinopathy, and macular degeneration will be discussed in later chapters.

When light strikes the rod and cone cells, it generates electrical impulses, which are transmitted through retinal nerve fibres to the optic nerve. The optic nerves from the two eyes join at the base of the brain, and then go to the occipital lobe, at the very back of the brain, where we actually perceive vision. The image on the retina is actually upside down but the brain turns it over so that we see it right side up.

At birth, our eye development is not yet complete. During the first few months of life the macula is still not fully developed, so babies can only focus for a distance of a few feet. They see less sharply than an adult does. Gradually, vision improves, and the retina reaches full development at about three months. By four or five months, the movement of both eyes is better coordinated and distance vision has improved. However, our eyes develop and grow until we are about 18 years old.

T W O

Eye Examinations

Regular eye examinations are crucial for maintaining healthy vision and regular visits should be made to an eye specialist. This chapter will outline what you can expect when you do have your eyes checked. Children should have their eyes examined by an eye specialist shortly after birth to determine whether there are any congenital defects and whether the eyes are normally developed. If no problems are found, the eyes should be checked again at about the age of three, and then at the start of school. Normally, a physician following the growth and development of a child will automatically include an eye examination in all assessments.

Those lucky enough to have no problems with their vision should have their eyes checked every few years; those with vision problems may need more frequent exams. People over 40 should be screened every year or two for glaucoma. After age 65, annual exams are needed to screen for glaucoma, cataracts, and macular degeneration. (These conditions will be defined and described in detail in later chapters.)

Eye examinations can be carried out by either an ophthalmologist or an optometrist. The ophthalmologist is a medical doctor (MD) who has become a specialist in eye problems and eye surgery. An optometrist is specially trained and licensed to examine eyes to determine the presence of vision problems and to prescribe corrective lenses; an optometrist has a Doctor of Optometry degree (OD). The type of practitioner you seek out is a matter of personal choice, as optometrists perform many of the same diagnostic procedures as medical doctors (MDs). If they discover or suspect a medical problem that requires diagnosis or treatment, they will refer you to an ophthalmologist.

In either case, the eye doctor is armed with a vast array of equipment, though not all the instruments will be used for every exam. The visit will begin with an external inspection of your face, eyelids, and eyes in normal light with the aid of a flashlight. Next comes the visual acuity test, using the Snellen Chart. This is the familiar eye chart with the large E on the top followed by lines of letters of decreasing size. You read the smallest line possible, first with one eye and then with the other, and if you wear glasses you do the test both with and without them. The result of this test is described as a ratio such as 20/40 or 20/60, meaning that at 20 feet you only see what someone with normal vision would see at 40 or 60 feet (12 or 18 metres). The worse your vision, the higher the second number.

The pupils of your eyes will also be evaluated, using a small light source like a penlight flashlight, to ensure that they are equal in size and that they react properly to increases and decreases in light. Subtle changes in the reaction of the pupils can indicate potential neurological problems.

Next, the interior of the eye will be checked with a small hand-held ophthalmoscope. This instrument has a light source, an aperture or opening, and a rotating wheel with multiple lenses for focusing the image, which takes into account the eyeglass prescription of both the examiner and the patient. With this, the ophthalmologist or optometrist can examine the optic nerve, the blood vessels, the retina, and the choroid.

The ophthalmoscopic examination and the pupil check are not just performed by ophthalmologists. Most physicians and optometrists, as part of their exam, will check the pupils and look into the back or interior of the eye.

Errors in refraction are measured with either an autorefractor or a manual retinoscope. Refraction refers to the eye's bending of light so that the image is focused exactly on the retina. If the light is not refracted properly, the image is focused either in front of or behind the retina and we don't see clearly. To prescribe the appropriate lens, the doctor must determine the amount of error in the refraction of light.

Automatic refractors are now becoming more popular. You focus on an object in a target area within the refractor, and a scanning device calculates the focusing characteristics of your eye and prints out the findings. To refine that setting, a manual refractor is used; you peer through two openings while the doctor flips different lenses. You then decide which of two lens choices gives the better vision.

The slit lamp may also be used as part of a regular exam. This is a binocular microscope that projects a narrow, intense beam of light both on and into the eye. The doctor can then see a cross-section of various parts of the eye under very high magnification, to check the health of the tissue. The slit lamp can also be used while removing foreign particles like dust or eyelashes from the eye.

Depending upon your symptoms, your age, and the findings from these evaluations, many other tests can be carried out. The ophthalmoscope only lets the examiner see the central area (the macula and optic nerve) of the interior of your eye. To examine the peripheral area, the area off to the side of the eye, where retinal detachments often occur, an indirect ophthalmoscope must be used. This consists of a headband with a bright light source and a binocular viewing system. A condensing lens is held in front of the patient's eye and in line with the light source. A small depressor is used to push back parts of the sclera to allow examination of the peripheral retina and inspection for possible tears. The process is not painful.

A keratoscope can be used to project a series of concentric rings of light onto the cornea. If the cornea is healthy, the reflections should be smooth, regular, and symmetrical. Distortions in the reflections may indicate disorder of the cornea.

The glaucoma checks done for those over the age of 35 involve measuring the pressure within the eye. The process is called tonometry. An instrument called an air-puff tonometer bounces a small burst of air off the surface of the cornea. The pressure of the eyeball determines the speed at which the air puff returns to the observer, and the speed is measured in millimetres of mercury. The higher the pressure, the greater the speed. The more commonly used instrument is the Goldman tonometer. Using a small prism attached to a slit lamp on an anesthetized cornea gives the most accurate measurement of eye pressure.

Tears

Tears are produced in the lacrimal glands at the outside corners of the upper eyelids to clean and lubricate the eyes. But tear-drainage ducts can become blocked, causing continuously watery eyes; this requires treatment by an ophthalmologist. When the lacrimal glands atrophy, the person has "dry-eye syndrome"—this can be uncomfortable and can

Colour Blindness

Colour blindness is a fairly common inherited problem, occurring in about 10 percent of men but less than 1 percent of women. The most common form of colour blindness is the inability to tell red from green, and is determined by having you look at a page with in coloured symbols within different-coloured backgrounds. People who are colour blind confuse the images. In addition to inherited colour blindness, some disorders of the optic nerve and retina can also produce abnormal colour vision. Many jurisdictions test for colour blindness as part of the driver's licence process.

interfere with the use of contact lenses. Other symptoms include itching and burning.

Dry eyes can be assessed by the examiner by slipping a strip of special filter paper between the eye and the lower lid, leaving it for five minutes, and measuring the amount of wetting that takes place. This is called the Schirmer test. A topical anaesthetic should not be used since it adds fluid which can give a false test through measurement of the anaesthetic fluid rather than the individual's tear production.

With excessive tearing, it must be determined if there is poor drainage. The punctum or opening of the tear duct system located at the inner corner of the eyelid can be dilated and water can be injected through the system to unblock the obstruction.

The tests described above are all that most people ever experience in an eye examination. But although the examination may seem minor and straightforward, it's an important step in maintaining your health. Many non-eye problems can be revealed by their effects on the eyes. This is why, when you visit a doctor for a problem other than your eyes, he or she may spend time examining your eyes. The diagnosis of what is wrong with you may be confirmed by changes in your eyes.

The problems that can reveal themselves through eye symptoms are too numerous to list here, but here are some of the more common ones.

- *Tumours.* When light enters the eye and is transmitted through the optic nerve, the pupil reacts. If there is any growth that presses on the optic nerve, the transmission will be interfered with and the pupil will not constrict or dilate as it should. This may indicate the presence of a tumour. Loss of side vision, double vision, limited motion of the eyes, or swelling of the optic nerves can also indicate more serious problems with the brain.
- *An overactive thyroid* (hyperthyroidism) can result in bulging eyes (exophthalmos), upper lids higher than normal (eyelid retraction), infrequent blinking (thyroid stare), compression of the optic nerve (optic atrophy), abnormalities of the eye muscles, and inflammation of the cornea.
- *Liver diseases* such as cirrhosis and hepatitis may first be detected when the white sclera becomes yellow. This condition is known as jaundice. Night blindness may also indicate a liver problem, because of vitamin A deficiency.
- Many other *vitamin deficiencies* may show up in eye examinations. For example, vitamin C deficiency can result in increased haemorrhages of the eye.
- *Side effects of medications* may also appear. For example, cortisone can cause cataracts and increased pressure inside the eye (glaucoma).

Given the complexity of the eyes, the number of problems that can occur, and what the eyes can tell us about the state of our overall health, regular eye examinations are crucial.

THREE

Problems of Childhood

Three main eye conditions affect children and must be dealt with quickly to avoid serious permanent damage: infantile cataracts, strabismus, and amblyopia. There are also a number of common but much more minor problems.

Infantile Cataracts

About one baby in 10 000 is born with a severe cataract or clouding of the lens, which prevents light from focusing properly on the retina. These cataracts may be inherited or may result from the mother contracting German measles in the first 3 months of pregnancy. Exposure to radiation or the use of some drugs during pregnancy may also produce cataracts in the infant.

Today, the major cause of infantile cataracts is galactosemia. This results from the absence of an enzyme required to digest the galactose sugar in milk. As the blood-sugar level rises, blood sugar begins to seep into the lens, causing it to absorb ocular fluid and lose its transparency.

If the cataracts are not removed quickly, the result can be amblyopia, or lazy-eye syndrome, which is discussed later in this chapter. Sometimes the cataracts can be seen as white dots in the pupil, but if a child fails to react to large, colourful stimuli, cataracts should be suspected even if they can't be seen and an ophthalmologist consulted.

Blindness is a very real danger with infantile cataracts, and they should be removed as soon as the child is physically able to undergo the general anaesthetic. Removal of the cataracts is essentially the same as for adults (see Chapter Five). The child will only need to be hospitalized for about a day. The bandage is removed the day after surgery. A protective shield is worn over the eye at night for a short period after the bandage comes off. Contact lenses can be fitted after surgery to take the place of the removed lens. Any type of contact lenses can be used as long as the parents are able to insert them and take them out for the child. Of course, it is easier if the parents themselves use contacts.

Another technique is to sew a contact lens made from human-donor cornea (called an epikeratophakia lenticule) to the infant's cornea, either at the time the cataract is removed or one or two months later. Some eye surgeons prefer to replace the cataract lens with an intraocular lens implant (an IOL, or artificial plastic lens) at the time of the initial surgery. Epikeratophakia is discussed in detail in Chapter Four, and lens implants are dealt with in Chapter Five.

Strabismus and Amblyopia

About 4 percent of children develop strabismus, which is the inability to align both eyes on the same object. This condition, in its more severe form, is often referred to as a crossed or wandering eye. In some instances, the strabismus is caused by farsightedness (the inability to see close objects). If that is the case, the problem can be corrected with glasses.

The movements of the eye are controlled by six small muscles attached to each eye, and a number of tests are used to determine whether these muscles are working properly or whether the child may have strabismus.

The alignment and coordination of the eyes can be determined by covering one and then the other eye with the back of the hand or an occluder. An occluder is simply a round disk, large enough to cover the eye, on a handle about 20 cm long. The disk is alternately positioned over the two eyes while the patient stares at an object 6 m away. This alternating interrupts the fusion mechanism of the eyes—that is, the normal tendency for the eyes to be focused on one object. If there is a tendency for the eyes to be misaligned or crossed, the test will cause this to happen. Covering and uncovering one eye rapidly will also reveal misaligned eyes. Prisms can be used to measure the extent of the misalignment.

The eyes are capable of moving in all directions while remaining aligned with each other. By having the patient follow a small light or object, the doctor can determine if there are any problems with seeing in different directions—if, for example, one eye moves in all directions while the other one can't move in one specific direction. This test can be done even with very small infants.

In another test, the physician will have the patient stare at a white light while looking through a red lens placed over one eye. If the eyes are perfectly aligned the patient will see only one pink light, but if there is any misalignment a red light and a white light will be seen separately.

The Worth four-dot red/green glasses test requires the patient to wear glasses with a red lens on one eye and a green lens on the other, and look at an array of red, green, and white lights. If vision is absent in one eye, one colour will not be seen. If there is double vision, extra lights will be seen.

Depth-perception testing involves special 3D (three-dimensional) glasses and a series of three-dimensional objects. When both eyes are functioning properly, we have depth perception, which can be quantified according to the number of objects seen. People with poor muscle coordination may not see in 3D and will do poorly with the test.

Eye exercises, glasses, and eye drops to assist in focusing are first attempted to correct the problem, but if these do not work, surgery is required. Today, this is fairly simple. The six muscles that control the eye are easily accessible to the surgeon and there is minimal risk to vision from the operation. In 90 percent of children, the procedure is successful after several months.

The surgeon makes an incision through the conjunctiva and adjusts one or more muscles. If the eye is turned inward, a tight inner muscle can be cut and reattached farther back. A weak muscle can be tightened by shortening it and stitching the ends back together. Healing is quite rapid and normal activities can usually be resumed very quickly. Double vision sometimes results right after surgery but this corrects itself within a few weeks.

About half the children with untreated strabismus develop

amblyopia, or "lazy eye." In addition, amblyopia can result from infantile cataracts, extreme nearsightedness, farsightedness, or astigmatism, or from large differences between the prescriptions for the two eyes. Normally, the brain receives signals about an object from both eyes and puts them together into one picture. This gives us depth perception and the ability to see in 3D. But when the images from the two eyes differ significantly, one image is ignored by the brain and visual function does not develop normally. The brain circuits that process vision are not complete until about the age of six, so it is crucial to treat this condition before that age. If left untreated, amblyopia can become permanent.

In addition to alleviating the underlying cause of the problem (such as strabismus or cataracts), treatment includes putting a patch over the good eye. This forces the child to use the "lazy eye." Unfortunately, it can be difficult to get small children to wear an eyepatch for any length of time.

A small number of infants are born with congenital glaucoma or retinal macular conditions, both of which are normally associated with ageing. An explanation of these problems is given in Chapter Five.

Other common problems in children

Conjunctivitis ("pinkeye") makes the eye sore and inflamed, and often produces a discharge. It is not limited to children, but tends to be quite common among them. This condition is usually caused by an infection or an allergic reaction. Bacterial conjunctivitis normally produces a greenish-yellow pus discharge that may cause the eyelids to stick together. The viral form of conjunctivitis usually has a more watery discharge. If the cause is an allergy, the eye is often itchy and swollen.

The first line of treatment is to soak the child's eyes every few hours with a warm water compress. The child should also be seen by an ophthalmologist. Antibiotic drops or ointment will be prescribed if the problem is bacterial. If it is bacterial, it is highly contagious and other members of the family as well as playmates should take careful precautions to avoid infection.

Occasionally, a hair follicle or oil-secreting gland at the base of an eyelash becomes blocked and infected. The inflamed red pimple that forms is known as a *sty*, and is caused by bacteria. Soaking with hot compresses for about five minutes, four or five times a day, will increase blood flow to the area and force the pimple to come to a head and burst. Antibiotic eye ointment may also be prescribed.

A common problem among newborns is *blocked tear ducts* that prevent the proper drainage of tears from the eyes into the nose. An overflow of tears will be seen and the lashes may be stuck together after sleep. If the problem is caused by too much mucus formation or the failure of the tear duct to open completely at birth, it often corrects itself after a few months. Gentle massaging of the duct near the nose may help speed up the opening process. If the condition has not improved by the age of about six months, the ducts may have to be opened surgically, by a small probe placed through the ducts under general anaesthesia.

F O U R

Refraction and Vision

Refractive Errors

As we said earlier, our vision depends on the refraction, or bending, of light. When rays of light pass through the transparent cornea and lens of the eye, they change direction. If the refraction is perfect, the light

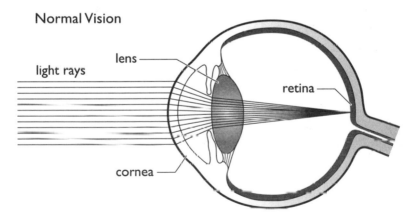

Normal Vision

light rays

lens —

retina —

cornea —

In normal vision, the light rays are bent as they pass through the cornea. Minor adjustments are made as the light passes through the lens so that they converge on the cornea and we see clearly.

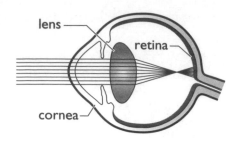

Myopia (nearsightedness)

rays come together or converge exactly on the retina and produce a clear but inverted image of whatever we are looking at. If the rays do not converge exactly on the retina, the result is poor vision: myopia, hyperopia, astigmatism, or presbyopia.

Myopia, or nearsightedness, is the inability to see clearly at a distance. As the diagram illustrates, the rays of light are bent too much and they converge at a point in front of the retina. Beyond this point, they begin to diverge again, so the image is scattered when it hits the retina and vision is blurred. However, objects that are close may be seen clearly.

In the case of *hyperopia*, the curvature of the cornea is a little too flat or the eye is smaller than normal, so that the

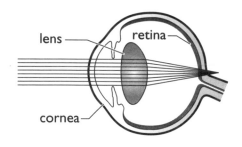

Hyperopia (farsightedness)

light rays have not yet converged when they reach the retina. As a result, close images are blurred but the individual can see things at a distance. The condition is commonly referred to as farsightedness. This problem occurs frequently in newborns and young children but lessens as the eye grows and matures.

Astigmatism can also affect our vision, by itself or in combination with one of the above conditions. Astigmatism occurs when the cornea or the lens is irregular, and is football-shaped rather than round. As a result, light rays converge at two different focal points in the eye, rather than at one point on the retina. The result is a distortion of vision.

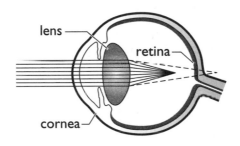

Astigmatism (distorted vision)

Presbyopia is another form of farsightedness. Although much refraction is done by the cornea, some of the refraction necessary to see objects at close range is performed by the lens of the eye, which can change shape depending upon the distance away of the item being looked at. With age, there is a gradual stiffening of the lens and the ciliary body (which contains the muscles that control the lens). This condition is known as presbyopia, and it reduces the ability to focus on near objects.

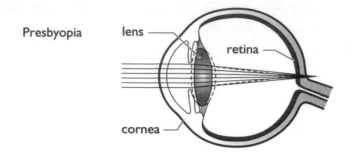

With advancing age, the lens is less flexible, and light rays from nearby objects focus behind retina instead of on it.

Presbyopia usually begins about age 40, and even people who never required glasses begin to find that they cannot read without them. Nearsighted people develop the problem a little later, since myopia compensates for presbyopia to some degree.

Causes of Refractive Error

It is interesting and baffling that about 50 percent of the population require glasses because of refractive errors. This implies that the shape of the cornea or the size of the eye is flawed in half the population. No other part of the body has such a poor record.

We know that whether people need glasses or not depends partly on heredity, but often theories about why some people are myopic or hyperopic are controversial. It has been suggested that myopia is aggravated by excessive reading or close work—in other words, that it's an affliction of civilization and relates directly to the literacy rate of society. During the

Renaissance, wearing glasses was considered a mark of learning. A few centuries ago, when fewer people could read, myopia was not as common. Today, children focus from an early age on visual points close to the eye, such as books and television. Also, living indoors limits the times that the eye must focus on distant objects. As the eye develops it retains the shape it has developed for nearsighted focusing, and myopia results.

One study among the Inuit found that older people who had not gone to school had no problems with myopia, but that their children, who went to school, did develop the condition. In addition, once adults started going to school, many of them became myopic. This observation led to the theory that disabling the focusing mechanisim of the eye with atropine (belladonna) drops might stop the development and progression of myopia. Studies to prove this theory have been inconclusive.

In the 1950s, it was learned that myopic children showed a more irregular growth pattern and earlier maturity than those with normal vision. The rate of myopia development correlated with growth spurts. It was also observed that children who ate little protein had a greater degree of myopia than children who ate more.

In one study, schoolchildren with myopia who were about equal in health and social level were divided into two groups. One group was given 10 percent of their caloric intake from protein, while the other group ate normally. The children on the high-protein diet had a slower progression of nearsightedness. These results have been replicated in young rabbits, but we still don't know if increased protein actually slows down the progression of myopia.

A History of Visual Correction

People have been trying to correct poor vision since the days of the Babylonian leader Hammurabi, almost 4000 years ago. His famous code of laws permitted people with "infirm eyes" to use aids to vision, but we don't know what these were.

Scientists and scholars throughout history have struggled to understand the mechanism of sight, and have experimented with magnification and refraction. In the eleventh century, the Islamic scholar Alhazen concluded that the optic nerve carried signals from the eye to the brain. A Polish scientist named Vitello was the first European to write a book on optics; he found that striking a convex (outward-curving) surface brings rays of light together while striking a concave (inward-curving) surface causes the rays to diverge.

Up until about the seventeenth century, anyone who needed glasses chose a pair by simple trial and error, since it was not possible to measure the refractive error. As knowledge of the physiology of the eye and refraction advanced, different-shaped lenses could be produced. In 1604, the German astronomer Johannes Kepler was able to define myopia. In 1793, the English physicist Thomas Young first described astigmatism, and in the mid 1800s the Dutch ophthalmologist Franciscus Cornelis Donders defined hyperopia.

In 1827, the English astronomer Sir George Airy, who suffered from astigmatism, invented a cylindrical lens to correct that condition. To grind lenses to a common standard, some form of measurement was required to denote the lenses' power. That standard measurement, which is still used today, was developed in France in 1872 by Monoyer, and is known as the dioptric system.

How Lenses Work

A concave (or minus) lens is required to correct myopia, while a convex (or plus) lens corrects hyperopia. As the power (curvature) is increased in either lens, the focus of light is further shortened or lengthened. With the appropriate lens the light will focus on the retina as it should. In the dioptric system, the power of a lens needed to correct hyperopia is expressed as a number from +1 to +20. The power of a lens for myopia is expressed as −1 to −20. Over 5 diopters in correction is considered high. Correction for astigmatism is built into lenses for myopia and hyperopia. Since the eye is not perfectly round in astigmatism but distorted in one direction, the lens distorts to the other direction to balance.

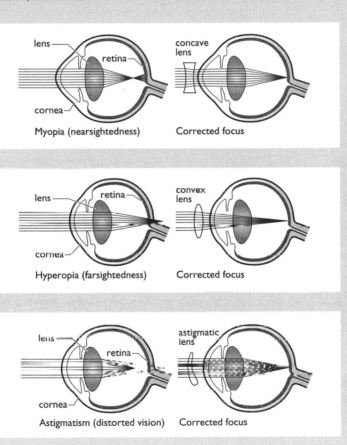

lens · retina · cornea
Myopia (nearsightedness)

concave lens
Corrected focus

lens · retina · cornea
Hyperopia (farsightedness)

convex lens
Corrected focus

lens · retina · cornea
Astigmatism (distorted vision)

astigmatic lens
Corrected focus

The idea for bifocals—glasses that correct myopia with the top half of the lens and have a different lens in the bottom for reading—was first conceived by Benjamin Franklin. By putting two separate lenses together, he could correct both myopia, and the presbyopia of advancing years, with a single pair of glasses.

Visual Correction Today

These days we have eight methods of correcting refractive errors:

- glasses
- contact lenses
- orthokeratology
- radial keratotomy (RK)
- photorefractive keratectomy (PRK)
- keratomileusis
- automated microlamellar keratotomy
- epikeratophakia

Glasses
It is now possible to purchase many different types of lenses and combinations of lenses. In addition to simple corrective lenses, there are bifocals, trifocals, blended bifocals, progressive-add lenses, and occupational lenses.

The most common bifocals are flat-tops, in which the reading portion of the bottom of the lens extends only partway across. Another style, the "executive" lens, has the reading portion all the way across the bottom, and is used by people who do a lot of reading and close work. Trifocals have three different focusing zones: the top portion is used for viewing distances, the middle portion is used for an intermediate zone (arm's length), and the bottom portion is used for reading (from 20 to 50 cm away).

Blended bifocals have the junction between the two segments polished so it's not evident that the person is wearing bifocals. This may result in an area of some distortion, which can be distracting for the user. Progressive-add lenses avoid this distortion while still concealing the fact that the individual is using bifocals. The top and bottom parts of progressive-add lenses are for distance and reading, respectively, but between these two the prescription changes gradually, in a series of steps. As a result, there are a number of focal points, allowing for clear vision at all distances.

Occupational lenses are designed for people with particular jobs or hobbies. An additional focal segment is added at the top of the lens so that near objects can be seen when the person is looking up. These lenses are sometimes needed by mechanics, electricians, and so on. Also people who spend a great deal of time at computer terminals can have an intermediate zone built in to facilitate their work.

If you don't have myopia but you need reading glasses, it's possible to purchase a pair in a drugstore. These are quite inexpensive but they are only suitable if both eyes require the same prescription. If that is not the case, your reading glasses have to be made by an optician for your specific needs.

It's very important that glasses be the right proportion for your face, because the optical centres of the two lenses must line up with the pupils. If they don't, vision can be uncomfortable or double vision can result. The frame must also be properly tilted, with the top portion a little farther away from the eye than the bottom part.

Glasses are still probably the most common method for correcting visual defects, and they are certainly the easiest and safest to use. But anyone who wears glasses knows the problems involved. Glasses get dirty, glasses get misplaced. Glasses tend to cut down peripheral vision—that is, the frames block part of our vision to the left and the right. They can also be a problem in rainy weather; not only do the lenses get rain or snow on them, but also they often fog up when we come in out of the cold. Even with the wide choice of designer frames available today, many people consider that glasses detract from their appearance. With the new shatterproof plastic lenses, glasses are safer than they used to be, but they still make it difficult to engage in a lot of sports.

For these and other reasons, alternatives have long been sought.

Contact Lenses

The oldest and most common alternative to glasses is the contact lens. Contacts are thin lenses that are worn right on the surface of the eye, over the cornea, floating on the eye's natural moisture. The first experimental contacts were developed in 1887, by a German physiologist, A.E. Fick, but they were not very successful.

In 1938, the development of a new plastic revolutionized contact lenses and their use became much more common. The lenses could be worn much or all of the day, but were removed at night. In 1958, bifocal lenses made their appearance, and in 1970, "soft" contacts entered the marketplace. Today, we have extended-wear disposable contact lenses that can be worn for two or three days and thrown away, lenses that will correct astigmatism, and even lenses that will change your eye colour.

Contacts have provided users with a great deal of freedom. They don't detract from appearance, they make it easier for people to engage in sporting activities, they help the extremely myopic person find the soap in the shower, and the extended-wear lenses let people see the time on the alarm clock when they wake up in the morning.

Today there is little difference between hard and soft lenses. Like other parts of the body, the cornea needs oxygen to survive. Initially, the soft lens let more oxygen through and so could be worn longer than the hard lens. However, hard lenses are now gas-permeable and also let oxygen through. Choosing hard versus soft is often a matter of comfort more than anything else. Bifocal and disposable lenses are soft. But soft lenses can't be used to correct significant astigmatism, because this requires a special "toric" lens that is weighted so that the astigmatism correction always stays in the same axis.

Extended-wear lenses that could be worn for up to a month were in vogue recently, but are no longer recommended. These lenses reduced the oxygen flow so much that about 5 percent of wearers developed severe corneal ulcers. Today, disposable lenses are quite popular. Length of wear for disposable lenses is controversial and is constantly changing. Many physicians and contact lens specialists, however, do recommend strongly that these contacts be removed every night.

The proper fitting of contacts is crucial for safe and comfortable wear. After a thorough eye exam and medical history, the curvature of the cornea is carefully measured using a keratometer. Next, a trial lens is placed on the cornea and left for about fifteen minutes, so that it can settle into place. The eye is then examined with the slit lamp to evaluate the suitability and fit. If hard lenses are being prescribed, fluorescein drops are used to further assess the fit. The lens should be wellcentred and should move slightly with each blink.

With the proper lenses in place, the person is given a wearing schedule that permits gradual adaptation. Any problem with irritation, tearing, redness, decreased vision, or pain should be reported immediately. At a re-examination within a few weeks, visual acuity is checked again and the fit is verified. The patient's wearing time is increased to the maximum, and appropriate follow-up examinations are suggested.

Although contacts free the wearer from the bother of glasses, they can require a considerable amount of care. The lenses must be cleaned and sterilized regularly and the person must practise good hygiene. For some people, these activities are bothersome and time-consuming.

There are also more health risks associated with contacts than with glasses. No matter how good contacts are, you are still putting a foreign object onto the cornea for a long time each day. Irritation, damage, and infection are potential problems that should be watched for. People who wear contacts should have their eyes checked regularly (usually once a year) and should stop wearing the lenses whenever irritation occurs.

Not everyone can use contacts. People with bad allergies may find that their eyes are so irritated by airborne allergens that the lens becomes intolerable. A small percentage of people suffer from dry-eye syndrome and the lack of moisture in their eyes makes it difficult or impossible for them to wear contacts.

In one recent study, it was found that between 10 and 20 percent of contact-lens wearers suffered allergy symptoms caused by their lenses or the cleaning solutions. The lenses of allergy-prone people quickly become coated with a film of proteins, particles of makeups, lipids, mucus, and microorganisms that add to the symptoms. A study of 855 patients found that those with positive allergy tests had double the rate of itching, tearing, burning, and redness compared with non-allergic users.

People with these problems should be meticulous about lens cleaning, and should use disinfecting solutions that are free of preservatives. They may find rigid lenses most suitable as they are more easily cleaned, but disposable lenses can also be helpful. Certainly, extended-wear lenses are no longer recommended.

Even if you have no unusual problems with your eyes, proper hygiene is crucial. Hands should be washed thoroughly before inserting or removing lenses. If you use makeup, make sure that it is not old, as the makeup can easily become contaminated with bacteria. Do not use someone else's makeup. Makeup, particularly mascara, should also be applied after the lenses are inserted.

Unless you have disposable lenses that can be tolerated for up to 72 hours, your contacts should be removed every night and cleaned thoroughly. There are numerous products on the market for cleaning and storing lenses and your contact lens specialist will recommend a system for you. However, you should never wet the lens with saliva, tap water, or saline solutions made from saline tablets. You run the risk of causing an infection or corneal ulcer due to bacteria or the particularly dangerous *acanthamoeba fungus.*

No matter what cleaning and care system is used, you will be using some form of daily cleaner, a saline solution and a storage solution. You should ensure that the container used to store the lenses is quite clean. Sometimes periodic protein removal is required in addition to the daily routine, as both protein and lipids or fat molecules can become coated on the contacts.

Because of this build-up, contacts should be replaced on a fairly regular basis. Your contact lens specialist will recommend periodic appointments to check the lenses. Finally, a current pair of prescription glasses should be kept on hand for those times when your eyes are sore or you have a cold and the lenses irritate.

Orthokeratology

A more dramatic use of hard contact lenses is to change the cornea so that glasses or full-time contact wear will no longer be required. This therapy is called orthokeratology.

This use for contacts was discovered by accident. Two Beverly Hills optometrists who specialized in prescribing hard contacts, Stuart Grant and Charles May, became curious when some of their patients mentioned that their vision was getting better the longer they used contacts. One patient even told them that he was halfway to work in his car, and seeing perfectly, when he realized that he had forgotten to put his lenses in.

Grant and May realized that the contacts were working rather like the braces a dentist uses on teeth, gradually flattening the cornea so that the myopia became less pronounced. The cornea is made of very pliable tissue, so this reshaping is not difficult to achieve. They developed a system using a series of different lenses, of less and less curvature, to gradually flatten the cornea more and more.

A considerable correction of myopia can be achieved with this method. Once the maximum effect is obtained, a retainer lens must be worn for short periods of time to prevent the cornea from slipping back to its former myopic state. The length of time this retainer must be worn varies with the individual. Some people wear them for a few hours a day, while others only need them a few times a week. Without this follow-up, the myopia will return.

Long-term monitoring has been done and patients have experienced no problems or side effects. However, once the patient stops using the retainer lens, the myopia returns to its former level. The system offers no permanent solution to myopia.

In addition, the amount of improvement possible with "orth K" is limited. It is not recommended for people with more than a −4 correction, as the eye will only improve by only 2 diopters. But for permanent correction of refractive errors, new surgical techniques are becoming available.

Radial Keratotomy (RK)
In 1972, a young boy in Moscow fell off his bicycle, shattered his spectacles, and lacerated his cornea. He was brought to the hospital and his eye was treated and bandaged. When the bandages were removed, he discovered that he could see without his glasses. The doctor who treated him, S.N. Fyodorov, realized that the radial pattern of the lacerations had flattened the cornea, reducing the boy's myopia. The result is radial keratotomy, a surgical correction that has been used on over a million myopic patients around the world.

This method is actually the second attempt to correct myopia by surgically altering the cornea. In 1939, a Japanese surgeon, Dr. Sato, developed an operation that he was convinced would end the need for glasses in Japan forever. His surgery involved flattening the cornea by making incisions on both the front and the back of it. These operations were successful initially, but over time problems began to appear. When the inside of the cornea was cut, a large number of vital cells were seriously damaged, allowing fluid to enter the cornea in abnormal amounts. This resulted in a gradual degeneration of the cornea, leading to blindness in a number of cases.

Fyodorov spent 3 years perfecting his surgery on animals, and performed his first human surgery in 1975. In the late 1970s the operation was first performed in Canada by Dr. Marvin Kwitko and in the United States by Dr. Leo Bores. In 1981, the U.S. National Eye Institute initiated PERK (Prospective Evaluation of Radial Keratotomy), a 5-year clinical study that evaluated 450 RK patients from 1981 to 1984. The conclusion, reported at the annual meeting of the American Academy of Ophthalmology in November 1984, was that radial keratotomy was safe and effective. The safety of this operation was also based on experience with corneal transplant operations, where a circular penetrating incision is made. Since transplant patients retain good vision and healthy corneas for a lifetime, it seems reasonable that the linear incisions of RK will achieve similar satisfactory results.

In radial keratotomy, four or more cuts are made in the cornea with a diamond scalpel. The cuts are made from the centre of the cornea to the outer edge, and the depth of the incisions depends on how much the cornea must be flattened to correct the refraction of light. More than four cuts are made if greater correction is required, but there is a limit to how much the cornea can be flattened. Results beyond about –9.0 diopters are usually not possible. Some degree of correction for astigmatism of up to 4 diopeters is also possible.

The surgery is carried out on one eye at a time, and only after very careful measurement of the thickness of the cornea. A topical (local) anaesthetic is used for the surgery, although in some cases the eyelids may also be frozen for further relaxation. The operation only takes about 20 minutes, but additional cuts may be required at a later date if the desired result has not been achieved.

After surgery, the eye is covered with a patch, and antibiotic drops (and sometimes anti-inflammatory drops) are used for a few days. Follow-up visits are arranged periodically in the first year, and then annually. The second eye is done once the first eye has stabilized and proper results have been achieved, usually four to six weeks later.

Complications are rare but possible, and the procedure is fully discussed with the patient before surgery, so that he or she is aware of the potential outcomes, the time required to achieve maximum benefit, and the side effects that may be experienced.

Some loss of effect is normal after surgery, as the cornea tends to regress slightly to its original shape. To compensate for this, the surgeon may overcorrect so that when the cornea heals it regresses to normal vision. In some cases the cornea does not revert far enough to eliminate this overcorrection, and reading glasses may be required. In other cases, astigmatism may be created by the surgery, if the cornea does not heal symmetrically. This astigmatism is usually too slight to require correction, but if it is more than expected, further surgery may be required.

About 85 percent of the people who undergo RK attain 20/40 vision or better, and about 30 to 35 percent attain 20/20 vision. People with 20/40 vision do not require corrective lenses while driving, but may need glasses to drive at night when the illumination is poor, or for watching movies or sporting events.

For those who still require some slight correction after surgery, it should be pointed out that contact lenses can't be worn for about 3 months, to give the cornea time to heal. In addition, contacts may be a little more difficult to fit and to tolerate, due to the changed shape of the cornea. Gas-permeable lenses will be the most appropriate.

Most people experience some side effects, but in almost all cases these clear up within 3 to 9 months. The eyes have an increased sensitivity to bright light for a short period; this is usually diminished as the cornea heals. "Haloes" around lights at night, an effect experienced by myopic patients when they take off their glasses or contacts, may be seen after RK. Night glare and "starburst" may be experienced, because extra fluid around the cuts causes light to scatter rather than pass directly through; this becomes worse at night as the pupil dilates to let more light in. Headlights from oncoming cars may also cause a starburst pattern. These problems diminish as the incisions heal, but in the meantime it may be necessary to use a mild constricting drop once a day, to close the pupil slightly.

Vision may fluctuate as the cornea heals and changes shape, being much better in the morning than in the late afternoon. This is probably due to variations in the eye pressure. Most people don't even notice these slight fluctuations, and they begin to clear up within months of the surgery. Night myopia may also be a problem, for reasons that are still not fully understood. During the day, when illumination is best, the pupil is smallest, so that light passes mostly through the flatter central part of the cornea. When illumination is poor, the pupil dilates to allow more light to pass through and the light enters mainly through the edges of the cornea. The curvature on the edges may be enough to cause a small amount of myopia. This phenomenon also appears in some people who have never had RK surgery, and it can be corrected by glasses or contacts worn only when it is dark.

The cornea is also weaker until the cuts have healed properly, so it's wise to take special precautions against any possible injury. Wearing racquetball goggles while engaging in work or sporting activities that could result in a blow to the eye is strongly recommended.

Most people who have radial keratotomy do so for occupational reasons, and the procedure is not covered by medicare programs, but some insurance companies cover some or all of the cost.

Photorefractive Keratectomy (PRK)

A promising new therapy for myopia called photorefractive keratectomy (PRK) is being tested with a new type of laser, the "cool" excimer laser. In the past, lasers have been used in medicine to cut tissue; light from the laser is absorbed mainly by the water in the tissue, resulting in an explosive reaction that cuts the tissue. The excimer laser, developed in the 1970s, produces a light in the far-ultraviolet portion of the spectrum, between 200 and 150 nanometres (thousand-millionths of a metre). The high energy of the light breaks the molecular bonds that hold tissue together. Because no heat is generated, there is no charring or damage to tissue, as there is with conventional lasers.

Unlike radial keratotomy, photorefractive keratectomy does not involve making incisions in the cornea. Instead, each pulse of the excimer laser removes a quarter of a micron (a micron is $\frac{1}{1000}$ of a mm) of tissue by vaporizing it. The amount to be removed is determined by the degree of myopia, and is precisely controlled by a computer.

The preparation and post operative care for PRK surgery is essentially the same as for RK surgery, and the conditions that the laser can treat are the same. But doctors hope the laser will also be able to treat hyperopia. The laser is presently more successful in correcting higher degrees of myopia.

Comparisons so far between RK and PRK suggest that they have an equal success rate. However, the side effects are different. With the excimer laser, a haze develops in the cornea about two months after treatment. This clears up in most cases, often with the use of cortisone eye drops. Also, decreased-contrast sensitivity is more pronounced at night, and this can affect driving.

A number of Canadian doctors are performing PRK, although start-up costs are high. The laser equipment costs about $500,000. Potential patients should be aware that this method is still under investigation in a 5-year clinical study by Health Canada. (Dr. Kwitko was chairman of the Advisory Committee on the Excimer Laser for Health Canada from 1990 to 1992 and formulated the protocol for the use of this laser on myopic and astigmatic patients in Canada.) By the end of 1995 the effects and results of these operations will be evaluated; the surgery will only be continued on an unlimited basis if the findings are favourable.

An evaluation of the first 350 patients who had PRK at the Institute for Laser Sight in Montreal showed that the procedure is very effective—80 percent of patients achieved 20/40 vision or better. The group with the greatest success had had –2 to –6 myopia; 90 percent of this group attained 20/40 vision or better, 80 percent of the –6 to –10 patients ended up with 20/40 while only 60 percent of the –10 to –15 group achieved 20/40 vision. Only 12 of the 350 patients were over-corrected, while the remaining group were undercorrected and were able to have a second treatment.

Keratomileusis and automated microlamellar keratotomy
Two other surgical techniques exist for people for whom RK is not appropriate, but they are much more complex.

Keratomileusis involves removing part of the cornea and re-sculpting it, much as an optician would do when grinding an eyeglass lens. The top portion of the cornea is removed, frozen, reshaped, thawed out, and sewn back in place. The procedure was originally developed by a Colombian surgeon, José Barraquer, in the early 1960s. It was adopted in the U.S. in the late 1970s, but did not become popular because of its difficulty, the expense of the equipment, and the training required.

Now, new equipment has made the procedure less complex. Freezing, which can damage delicate corneal tissue, is no longer required. The cornea is fixed in place by a suction ring and an instrument called a microkeratome cuts off the top portion, the dome of the cornea. The part that is removed is clamped to a shaping device while the microkeratome cuts away sections of the cornea. For myopia correction, the central part of the cornea is thinned to reduce curvature. For hyperopia, the peripheral portions are thinned. Once the resculpting is complete, the removed corneal part is sutured back in place.

A second new technique, automated microlamellar keratotomy, is based on the same concept. In this operation, the corneal dome is removed and then a second slice is removed (like cutting a salami), based on the amount of myopia or hyperopia; the corneal dome is replaced without the need for sutures.

The surgery is usually done under a local anaesthetic. Most potential complications are the same as for RK—that is, infection, perforations, undercorrection or overcorrection, and induced astigmatism. In addition, two other possible complications are unique to this operation.

When the top protective epithelial layer of the cornea is disturbed by injury, it begins to replace itself. As a result of

---

A Note about Lasers

The excimer laser is only one of many types of lasers that eye surgeons use. Indeed, the laser has become one of the most important pieces of ophthalmological equipment, and is used for treating many conditions.

Laser stands for Light Amplification by Stimulated Emission of Radiation, and the idea was first theorized by Albert Einstein in 1917. He hypothesized that under certain conditions, atoms or molecules could absorb light or other radiation and then be stimulated to shed their borrowed energy. During the 1950s, both Soviet and American physicists theorized about lasers, and in 1960 the first laser was built.

Lasers have a wide range of uses. They can be used to transfer photos and maps to printing plates, to find fingerprints on long-dead bodies, to weld metal, or to create 3D images. Simply put, an electrical current is used to disturb the electrons in a substance; when the atoms restabilize, tiny bursts of surplus energy called photons escape. A photon is the basic unit of light. The photons are manipulated by mirrors to generate more photons, which eventually escape in a beam of pure, concentrated light.

Common light from something like an ordinary lightbulb is a mixture of wave lengths, all going in different directions. Laser light, however, is coherent — it has only one wave length, and all the waves are moving in the same direction, in unison, so they reinforce each other. Because of that, a laser beam can go as far as the moon and then echo all the way back to earth.

---

the surgery, this epithelial layer may develop *between* the removed part of the cornea (the dome) and the rest of the cornea. Usually this tissue can be flushed out, but if this can't be done, then the outer part (the dome) of the cornea must be removed again and the underlying layers cleaned before the resculpted tissue is sewn back on. Also, no matter how much care is taken during the operation, it is possible for foreign particles to become trapped between the two parts of the cornea. If that happens, inflammation and opacities will occur. Again, the outer part of the cornea may have to be lifted so the particles can be removed.

The side effects of both techniques are also basically the same as for RK. With keratomileusis there may also be irritation of the stitches, or a suture may come loose and have to be removed.

Despite the complexity of this operation, results are usually quite good. Many people still need glasses or contacts, but they have a considerable reduction in their degree of myopia.

Epikeratophakia

For patients with a very high degree of hyperopia, a surgical treatment called epikeratophakia can be effective. It can also be used for people who have their lenses removed as the result of cataracts and who cannot, for some reason, have a plastic lens implanted.

This surgery, developed in the U.S. in 1980, involves sculpting donated corneal tissue into what is essentially a permanent contact lens. Before the operation, donor tissue is sculpted specifically for the patient, so that refractive error is eliminated. At first the donated tissue was frozen and then sculpted, but the freezing could damage the tissue. Now the excimer laser is being tried, to see if it can sculpt the tissue without the need for freezing.

During surgery, the outer corneal layer (epithelium) is removed and the surgeon makes a shallow groove around the cornea. The new tissue is placed over the cornea, tucked into the grooves, and sutured in place. Within a few weeks, the new tissue heals onto the eye and is covered by a new layer of protective epithelial cells.

Again, all possible complications and side effects that can occur with the other forms of surgery apply to epikeratophakia.

The one big advantage is that the operation is reversible; if there are serious problems, the grafted tissue can be removed. But there is a long healing process. It can take up to a year for the eye to stabilize and for the patient to see positive results. Also, when the operation is done on people with severe hyperopia, the results are rarely perfect. About three-quarters of patients will still require corrective lenses after this operation.

F I V E

Age-related Changes

T he most frequent age-related eye problem—the need for reading glasses—results from the lens becoming less elastic and less able to make minor adjustments. In addition, the cornea slowly begins to lose its inner protective cells, and may become thicker and more likely to scatter light. Also, the pupil becomes smaller with age, so that less light is admitted, and we require brighter lighting to see properly. You may find that the reading light beside your chair is no longer bright enough to let you read easily.

These changes may be annoying, but are relatively harmless compared with other serious problems that can occur as we age. These include cataracts, glaucoma, and macular degeneration.

Cataracts

As part of the ageing process, the crystalline lens begins to lose its clarity. This is referred to as a cataract. The loss of clarity

Normal Vision and Vision with Cataract

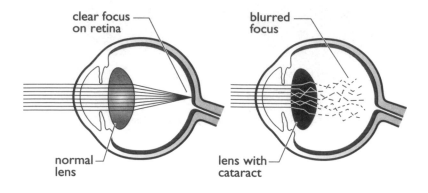

The hazy cataract prevents light from focusing on the retina.

causes hazy vision that may eventually prevent the person from seeing. Surgery for cataracts is the most frequently performed medical procedure in the U.S., and accounts for about 12 percent of the total medicare budget. In 1988 over one million lens implants were done in the U.S. and today the figure is over 1.5 million. Approximately $4 billion per year is spent in the United States on cataract removal. Slightly fewer procedures are done in Canada on a proportional basis.

Consider Roy, a man of 71 who had enjoyed good vision all his life. One day he noticed that the vision in one eye had become slightly blurred, and that when he drove into the sun the glare was almost disabling. As the blurring and glare became worse, Roy went to an ophthalmologist who noted that Roy's vision had declined from 20/20 to 20/40 and that there were some cataract developments in his lens. Roy was told to return for a checkup in 6 months. Over the course of that time, he noticed that he was having more difficulty driving, he was beginning to develop double vision, and he was having problems reading. His physician recommended surgery and made arrangements for him to enter the hospital.

The Causes of Cataracts

Until quite recently, cataracts were thought to be a natural part of ageing, as they develop in almost everyone over the age of 65. Now there is some evidence that cataracts result from a process known as free radical pathology. This chemical reaction is thought to be responsible for accelerating ageing, and may cause many of the degenerative diseases of ageing, such as arthritis and coronary heart disease.

A free radical is an oxygen molecule with an odd number of electrons. Normally, molecules have an even number of electrons, and this unpaired electron creates an imbalance leading to instability, violent reactivity, and destruction. The free radicals attack other molecules, damage them, and set off a chain reaction producing even more free radicals.

Chemical reactions that are a normal part of our metabolic processes produce a certain number of free radicals. We have natural defences to keep this process under control and to neutralize the free radicals when their usefulness is over. Several enzymes perform this function, as well as vitamins C and E, and beta carotene.

Unfortunately, environonmental agents may interfere with this built-in control system and increase the activity of the free radicals. As well, lifelong exposure to ultraviolet light seems to promote cataract formation. Dietary fats and alcohol have the same effect. A number of studies have demonstrated a link between diets rich in the anti-oxidant vitamins and a decreased risk of cancer and heart disease.

Smoking increases the number of free radicals, and may increase the risk of cataracts, and that risk likely grows with the number of cigarettes consumed. In a study of 17,000 male physicians and 69,000 female nurses, there was a strong link between smoking and cataracts—the heavier smokers had a greater risk. Scientists at Johns Hopkins Medical Centre in Baltimore have concluded that up to 20 percent of cataracts may be attributed to smoking.

The nurses in the study who had taken vitamin C supplements for ten years or more had a much lower risk of cataracts. Eye fluids are rich in vitamin C, possibly as a protection for the delicate eye tissues. A high intake of spinach was also found to be associated with a decreased risk of cataracts.

Trauma can also induce cataracts. If the lens is pierced, it may become cloudy, or the cataract process may be speeded up by a physical blow. Secondary cataracts can also result from diseases such as diabetes mellitus—patients with diabetes are three to four times more likely to develop cataracts. Other eye problems such as glaucoma can also increase the risk, as can the use of corticosteroid medications.

Learning to prevent or slow down cataract formation would not only benefit our ageing population, but also bring about a tremendous saving for our health care system. The U.S. National Institute of Health estimates that if the onset and development of cataracts could be delayed 10 years, cataract surgery could be reduced by 50 percent. That would bring about a significant saving.

Cataracts can form in any or all parts of the lens. In older people, it is the nucleus (innermost portion) of the lens that tends to become opaque. This is known as a senile or nuclear cataract and can begin as early as age forty, although it is most common in the late sixties. If a cataract forms on the outer edge

A Brief History of Cataract Treatment

Ancient India was the birthplace of the cataract operation, but word of it spread to the eastern Mediterranean after the Indian expedition of Alexander the Great. The first written record of the operation in Europe is in the works of the Roman writer Celsus about AD 30.

The technique was called couching, or needling. The lens was essentially pushed out of the area of the pupil and into the vitreous, where it remained. Some vision was restored; light could pass through the pupil unobstructed, but the focusing capability provided by the lens was gone, and images did not converge properly on the retina. (The cataract lens was left intact because early physiologists didn't understand its purpose. The lens was considered the central organ of vision, and to damage it when it was being pushed out of the way, it was believed, would destroy vision.)

In 1748, the French physician Daviel developed a method for extracting the lens rather than pushing it into the eye. Then in 1776 an Italian oculist, Tandini, came up with the idea of replacing the removed lens with an artificial one. He attempted an implant in 1795 but, given the materials and instruments of that time, was not successful.

of the lens, it is less likely to interfere with vision. Gradually, vision becomes distorted and blurry, with an increasing yellowish haze. As the cataract spreads, there will be difficulties with colour perception and deteriorating night vision. Vision may be worse in extreme brightness or glare, and there is a loss of depth perception. The person may need to change corrective lenses more frequently.

The development of modern cataract surgery

During the Second World War, Dr. Harold Ridley, a surgeon in the Royal Air Force, treated pilots who had had plastic particles imbedded in their eyes when the canopies of their planes were shattered. Some of these particles caused eye irritation— but some did not.

Ridley discovered that particles from the Spitfire fighter

canopy could remain in the eye without causing any permanent problems, while pilots with the same injury from other aircraft developed severe reactions. He learned that a different material was used to make the Spitfire canopy, a plastic known as PMMA (polymethylmethacrilate), and concluded that this plastic would be ideal as a lens replacement because it didn't react with body tissues.

After the war, Dr. Ridley worked on development of the plastic lens with some success. However, this was before the era of microsutures and the surgical microscopes needed for microsurgery. As a result, the technique was stopped. Dr. Ridley visited North America in the late 1950s and operated in several cities. Some doctors continued to perform his technique but the success rate was not high. The idea was ahead of its time.

By the late 1960s, surgical techniques had been developed by other eye surgeons, such as Cornelius Blinkhorst of Holland, to the point where the removal and replacement of the lens was safer and more effective. Dr. Kwitko trained with Dr. Blinkhorst in 1968 and performed the first successful series of implant operations in Canada in 1969. Today, it is a standard technique and a relatively simple operation.

Cataract surgery today
The treatment of cataracts is now almost miraculous; indeed, the surgery can usually be done as an outpatient procedure. The only remedy is replacement of the lens, and about 99 percent of cataract patients pick this option. Removal is crucial, because with a cataract in place it is very difficult for the ophthalmologist to see into the eye to check for the other common problems of ageing. Research with drugs to prevent or retard cataract formation holds great promise, but so far none have been successful.

About an hour before the surgery, the patient is given a sedative, and eye drops to dilate the pupil and anaesthetize the eye. This is supplemented by injections of anaesthetic under the lower eyelid to freeze the eye and the area surrounding it. A microscope is focused on the eye, and a retractor keeps the eyelid open. Three different methods are used to remove cataracts:

- intracapsular surgery
- extracapsular surgery
- phaco-emulsification.

In *intracapsular surgery*, all three parts of the lens—the nucleus (the innermost part), the cortex (the outer portion), and the capsule—are removed. Until the mid 1970s this was the procedure of choice, but it is now performed only in special cases, for example, a dislocated cataract.

The surgeon begins by making a semicircular cut halfway around the edge of the cornea, to have enough room to remove the entire cataract. A cold probe, called a cryoprobe, is placed on the cataract to freeze it so it can be lifted out. A small hole is then made in the iris to allow the flow of aqueous humour through the pupil; a blockage could cause secondary glaucoma. The incision is closed with about seven to ten stitches and antibiotic is injected under the conjunctiva to prevent infection.

The advantage of removing the entire cataract is that there is no chance of a secondary cataract developing in the portion of the lens that remains. The disadvantage is that in a few cases the frozen lens pulls some of the vitreous jelly out with it. This can lead to retinal detachment, swelling of the retina, and glaucoma, in less than 5 percent of the operations.

"Ripe" Cataracts

Before the development of intracapsular surgery, cataract surgery could not be performed until the cataract was entirely opaque, or "ripe," and hard enough to be manipulated. This meant that people had to endure long periods of declining vision before they could be helped. Nowadays cataracts can be treated as soon as they present a problem.

Another disadvantage is that because of the stitches around the eye, a month-long period of inactivity is required while the incision heals.

Extracapsular surgery involves leaving the posterior or back part of the capsule but removing the anterior or front part and the nucleus. Picture the lens as an M & M candy with the hard shell being the capsule and the inside the nucleus. With this procedure, the front half of the shell and the inside are removed, leaving the hard posterior surface.

The advantage of this method is that it helps to prevent retinal detachment and macular edema, or swelling of the retina. It also decreases the chance of some of the vitreous jelly being pulled out with the cataract. As well, the posterior part of the capsule can be used to support the implanted lens.

Because the posterior capsule is left, there is always the possibility that it too will become cloudy. A small hole can be made in the capsule to prevent this, but it can still happen. If the capsule does become cloudy later, it has to be opened at that time. This can be done quickly in the doctor's office, using a laser. The hole is the same size as the pupil so that if clouding does occur, it does not interfere with vision.

Phaco-emulsification is carried out with an ultrasonic needle that passes into the eye through a small incision. The needle vibrates at a high frequency, breaking the cataract into

Cataract Removal and Lens Insertion

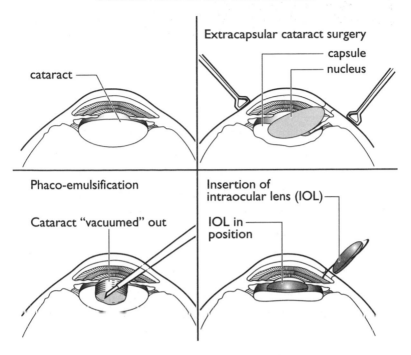

During extracapsular cataract surgery, the surgeon removes the nucleus of the lens but leaves the lens capsule. The next step is phaco-emulsification, where a "blender" type of device is inserted to break up the cataract and vacuum it out. The surgeon then slips a new plastic lens into place and positions it to replace the removed cataract lens.

particles that can be drawn out by suction, while leaving the posterior capsule intact. The big advantage of this method is that recovery is rapid, since only a very small incision is made and only one suture is required.

Now the eye is ready to receive its new lens.

Lens implants

Artificial implants have two main parts—the haptic, which holds the lens centred in place, and the optic, the actual lens substitute.

The design and power of the implant is carefully selected for the particular patient. The doctor measures the curvature of the cornea and the length of the eyeball, and then calculates how much focusing power the implant requires to converge light on the retina for a clear image. The doctor may choose a lens that will leave the patient slightly nearsighted, so that weak glasses are needed for distance but not for reading. A new type of lens that allows both near and far sight is called the multifocal lens implant.

Lens implants are classified by their position within the eye. There are four basic types:

- the posterior chamber lens
- the anterior chamber lens
- foldable lenses
- iris clip lenses.

The *posterior chamber lens* is the one most commonly used today. The lens rests behind the iris and in front of the posterior wall of the capsule, which is left intact after surgery. These lenses provide excellent vision and are very safe.

The *anterior chamber lens* is inserted in the fluid-filled chamber in front of the iris and behind the cornea. This type is used only if the posterior capsule is damaged during surgery and will not support the lens implant, in which case a posterior chamber lens might fall back into the vitreous.

Once the nucleus and cortex, or outer portion, of the cataract are removed, the back part of the capsule is distended with a gelatin material of high molecular weight. This gelatin is designed to protect the delicate ocular tissues from damage when the implant is manoeuvred into place. The new lens is inserted into the eye, and guided behind the cornea and under the edges of the remaining anterior capsule. Once it is properly positioned, the gelatin inserted before and during implantation is drawn out of the eye by suction. Next, the pupil is constricted with a drug and the incision is sewn up.

Foldable lenses are used after the phaco-emulsification procedure, which can be performed through a tiny incision only three mm long. These lenses can be folded, inserted through the incision, and then unfolded inside the eye—rather like the "wall anchors" used to hang pictures on wallboard, which are inserted through a small hole and then snap open inside the wall.

Iris clip lenses are attached to the iris, but are rarely used today because they can become dislocated when the pupil dilates.

Implant results

An occasional complication with any implanted lens is lens slippage, or "subluxation," described as either "sunrise" or "sunset." This comes about when the posterior capsule and supporting zonules aren't strong enough to support the lens implant. The zonule holds the lens in place. If the implant slips up so that all the doctor can see is the bottom edge, it's described as a sunrise; if it slips down so that nothing is seen but the top edge, it's described as a sunset. Neither condition is painful, but if the partial displacement reduces vision, a second operation will be required.

Optimal vision may not come back completely for 6 to

8 weeks after a lens implant, because the sutures can't be removed until healing is well on its way. A new valve-like incision used by some surgeons requires no sutures, or at most one or two. This has reduced recovery time to a few days or perhaps 2 weeks.

As with other medical devices implanted in the body, the long-term safety of artificial lenses has been a concern. When implants were first used in Canada in 1967, they were not recommended for anyone under the age of 60, but since then concern about their safety has diminished. Today they are used in people as young as 45, and even in children.

After lens-implant surgery
After surgery, the patient will feel a number of sensations. The most common is the feeling that there is something in the eye. This results from the presence of sutures and is a normal effect, but if the feeling is very irritating and persistent, it many mean a suture has come untied. It may also indicate a corneal abrasion (scratching), and if it doesn't clear up within several hours the surgeon should be notified.

A slight amount of increased tearing is also normal; this is associated with the sensation of something in the eye. If the tearing is excessive, and especially if the tears are pink, blood-tinged, or yellowish, the surgeon should be notified immediately.

There is always some increased sensitivity to light immediately after surgery, and some patients wear a patch or use sunglasses. If a patch is used, it is only required for a day and then sunglasses are used.

Frequently a bubble of air remains in the eye for a few days. It may be visible as a silver bubble moving around. This will clear up in three days at most.

Potential complications of implants

With all types of surgery, complications are possible. Serious infections occur once in every 10 000 cataract operations. The infection of a cataract operation produces extreme pain, sensitivity to light, and a swollen eyelid. The pain goes up into the top of the head, much like a toothache. There can be fever and the patient can feel very ill.

The pseudomonas germ is the most virulent, and this infection can destroy the eye in a matter of hours. This is quite rare, but no matter what type of germ infects the eye, hospitalization is required as quickly as possible. The surgeon will draw some fluid from the eye for culturing, to identify the bacteria, and the appropriate antibiotics will be given intravenously, orally, and by injection around the eye. In extreme cases, a vitrectomy is required; this is a surgical procedure where the vitreous jelly that contains the abscess is removed to prevent bacteria reaching the retina and causing blindness.

Even though infection is a remote possibility, it is why only one eye is operated on at a time. The chance of infecting both eyes simultaneously is very slight, but every precaution is taken.

Another possible complication is corneal edema, or swelling. If the patient has a diseased cellular layer in the cornea (called endothelial dystrophy), cataract surgery may cause further damage. Damaging these cells results in a thickening and whitening of the cornea and reduces the patient's vision. This usually lasts a few weeks and most often responds to intensive treatment with cortisone drops and injections. In less than 1 percent of cases it will not respond, and a corneal transplant may be necessary.

The pressure inside the eye may be elevated for several days after a cataract operation. This is a form of glaucoma, and usually responds to glaucoma therapy; the condition does not generally recur. Pre-existing glaucoma normally improves after cataract surgery, since the surgeon can combine a glaucoma procedure with cataract removal. In some instances, though, the glaucoma gets worse, and the patient experiences haziness of vision, pain, and even violent vomiting. Testing will indicate that pressure in the eye is high. Surgery is not usually required as medical management will alleviate the pressure. In these instances, the patient may have to use medication permanently.

In about 2 percent of cataract operations, the macula—the central part of the retina, which is crucial for reading—is swollen for as long as 2 years after surgery. This is called cystoid macula edema (CME) and it results in a considerable decline in vision. In most cases vision returns to normal within a couple of weeks, although it can take up to a year to clear up. It is very rare for vision to be permanently affected. Cortisone may be used to reduce the inflammation.

If, after surgery, you suddenly begin to lose your central vision, it is likely that you have macular edema. A fluorescein angiogram is carried out to determine this; fluorescein dye is injected into an arm vein and a picture is taken of the retina. If the macula is swollen, the dye leaks out and shows up in the photograph. Macular edema can occur even in the most uneventful cataract procedure.

In less than 1 percent of patients, a retinal detachment occurs after cataract surgery, usually in people who are highly myopic or who had a complication during surgery. The main visual symptom is a black cloud coming up from the ground or coming down from above. The condition is reparable, but the patient should be treated by an ophthalmologist as quickly as possible. Retinal detachments are discussed in Chapter Six.

People with diabetes or heart disease are susceptible to retinal haemorrhage from broken blood vessels. A haemorrhage can cause various degrees of vision loss, including complete blindness. It may also be associated with a rise in pressure within the eye. Immediate treatment is essential. Small haemorrhages in the conjunctiva of the eye usually clear without any effect on vision.

Sometimes the posterior capsule is torn during the cataract operation, and the surgeon is unable to remove all the soft cortex, or outer edge, and hard nucleus. If the material left is from the soft cortex, it will usually be absorbed by the normal healing process, and the reduced vision will improve in time. On rare occasions, particles of the hard nucleus fall into the back of the eye through the rip in the capsule. These will have to be removed later if the eye becomes inflamed.

Removal of cataracts does not always result in perfect vision. If a cataract is very dense, the surgeon can't see properly into the eye. It may turn out that other conditions that the surgeon was unable to determine before surgery will limit vision. This can be very frustrating for the patient, who sometimes incorrectly blames the surgeon for not doing a proper job.

For example, some patients suffer from amblyopia, or "lazy eye," and are not aware of it (see Chapter Three). Similarly, senile macular degeneration may go undetected because the surgeon can't properly examine the back of the eye through the cataract (see "Macular Degeneration," later in this chapter)

There is always a chance that the posterior capsule will begin to cloud up. If it does, the perfect vision the patient enjoyed after the surgery begins to fade and becomes hazy as it did when the cataract was forming. The remedy is fairly simple—the capsule is opened up with a laser in the doctor's office. The procedure is known as YAG (yttrium/ aluminum/garnet) laser capsulotomy and no convalescence is required afterwards.

Despite the potential complications and conditions that can influence the success of cataract surgery, more than 95 percent of patients find an improvement in vision and more than 90 percent obtain 20/40 vision or better. A high percentage have 20/20 vision without glasses. If the patient's vision does still require slight correction, this can be achieved with prescription glasses or contact lenses.

Cataract glasses

When both a patient's lenses have been removed because of cataracts, and artificial lenses have *not* been implanted, cataract glasses will be needed—they are known as aphakic glasses. Aphakic glasses cannot be used when cataract removal has been performed on only one eye and the other eye works properly, because the brain is unable to reconcile the two very different images. The solution is to use a special contact lens for the operated eye, or to cover one of the eyes with a patch. Aphakic glasses are only used after both eyes have been operated on but left without lens implants, or if the other eye has a dense cataract and poor vision.

Post-operative home care

After cataract removal, the patient needs advice about returning to his or her previous medical routine, particularly if it includes anticoagulant drugs or drugs to control blood pressure. These anticoagulant medications are stopped before surgery, and the ophthalmic surgeon may want to consult the patient's regular physician about how soon the usual drug routine should be resumed.

As well, the surgeon may prescribe drugs for post-surgical home use, and the patient should obtain them before surgery so there is no delay in starting them. Any caregiver the patient has should ensure that instructions for the use of medications are well understood, as the instructions are often in print that is too small for the patient to read.

Putting drops into the eyes can sometimes be a problem. This is an easy method:

1. The patient lies flat (without a pillow) on a bed or couch with the operated eye lightly closed.
2. Several drops are dropped into the recess near the bridge of the nose.
3. The patient blinks a few times and the eye drops flow naturally into the eye.

Protective plastic eye shields can be taped on from the forehead to the face, avoiding the jawbone. The easiest method is to stick the tape on the shield before putting the shield on the face. The cloth tape used in hospitals is often irritating; plastic or paper tape is better.

During waking periods, glasses should be used, and dark glasses are helpful against extreme sensitivity to bright light. Clip-on sunglasses can be used over regular lenses. Cleansing the eye with warm water and cotton balls or a washcloth helps to increase eye comfort. It is not necessary to use sterile cotton.

The person will be able to manage personal hygiene, cook simple meals, and do light housework. Help will be needed with shopping and most other work for a couple of weeks, help with heavy tasks will be needed for about 6 weeks. It is easy to forget the restrictions on bending, lifting, and straining, as there is no eye pain or discomfort when these actions are done, and numerous reminders may be needed. People recuperating from cataract surgery should *not* attempt heavy lifting jobs: they shouldn't lift the mattress to tuck in sheets, or hoist big garbage cans or vacuum cleaners. In addition, they should be careful not to poke their eye with the arm of their glasses as they put them on. They should have someone put away scatter rugs and change complicated furniture arrangements that increase the risk of slipping or bumping into things.

Glaucoma

Glaucoma has been called a "thief in the night," because it can creep up and destroy vision with minimal signs or symptoms. It is preventable, yet remains one of the leading reasons for blindness in North America.

Consider Frank's case. For a few months he had been noticing haloes around lights. At first he didn't pay much attention, but the condition became more severe. He had no eye pain, discomfort, or change in his vision, but as the halos grew more irritating he decided to see his eye doctor.

The doctor checked Frank's eye pressure and found that it was 32 mmHg in one eye and 28 mmHg in the other. (Normal pressure ranges between 8 mmHg and 22 mmHg.) A field-of-vision test was ordered and a "scotoma," an area of impaired vision that is characteristic of glaucoma, was detected. Open-angle glaucoma was diagnosed and Frank was put on eye drops twice a day. When the pressure remained above 22 mmHg, the medication was changed.

Despite the switch in medication, the pressure did not come down. The pressure remained high even after argon laser trabeculoplasty. Because of the severity of the glaucoma,

Chronic Open-Angle Glaucoma

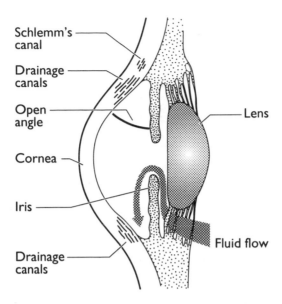

Schlemm's canal

Drainage canals

Open angle

Cornea

Iris

Drainage canals

Lens

Fluid flow

The space between the iris and cornea is open to allow the aqueous humour to drain away but there is a blockage in the drainage canal preventing this. This produces a build-up of pressure.

a trabeculectomy operation was performed. This brought Frank's eye pressure down to 15 mmHg. His haloes disappeared and the danger of doing permanent damage to his vision was averted, but he would have to remain on medication to keep the pressure controlled, and see his ophthalmologist regularly.

Patricia's case came on differently. She was 48 and in good health when she suddenly developed a sharp pain in her left eye while at a movie. At the same time she developed severe nausea, and went to the washroom, where she vomited. As

Acute Closed-Angle Glaucoma

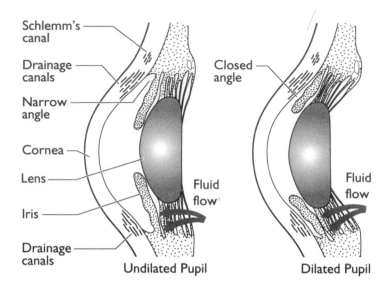

Schlemm's canal

Drainage canals

Narrow angle

Cornea

Lens

Iris

Drainage canals

Closed angle

Fluid flow

Fluid flow

Undilated Pupil

Dilated Pupil

When the pupil is undilated, as it would be in bright light, the angle between the iris and the cornea is narrow. When the pupil dilates in the dark, in order to allow more light to enter, the angle between the iris and cornea becomes closed. This restricts the flow of aqueous humour and causes a build-up of pressure.

the eye pain and nausea persisted, she went to the nearest emergency room.

After Patricia was examined by the attending physician, the ophthalmologist on call was summoned. The pressure in her left eye was 57 mmHg and she was diagnosed with acute closed-angle glaucoma. She was admitted to hospital and put on intravenous manitol fluid and pilocarpine drops, and her eye pressure dropped back to normal.

The following day, the ophthalmologist performed a laser iridectomy on Patricia's eye, and her glaucoma was cured. A

The Human Eye

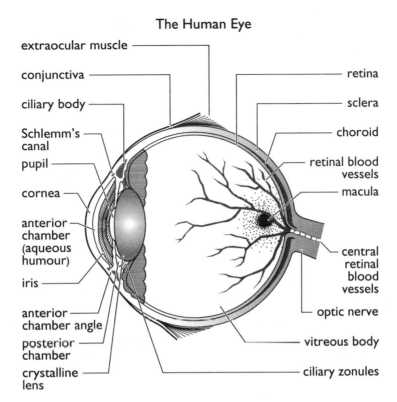

extraocular muscle

conjunctiva

ciliary body

Schlemm's canal

pupil

cornea

anterior chamber (aqueous humour)

iris

anterior chamber angle

posterior chamber

crystalline lens

retina

sclera

choroid

retinal blood vessels

macula

central retinal blood vessels

optic nerve

vitreous body

ciliary zonules

few weeks later, the surgeon repeated the laser treatment on her other eye, since acute glaucoma of this type commonly appears in both eyes.

What is glaucoma?

Glaucoma is the name of a group of disorders that result from excessive pressure within the eye. This increase in pressure, if untreated, can cause destruction of the optic nerve and produce blindness. The front of the eye is filled with a clear fluid (aqueous humour) that helps nourish the lens, cornea, and iris. This fluid is continually produced by the ciliary body (located

Glaucoma Damage

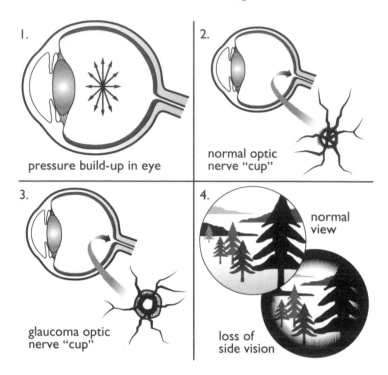

When the aqueous humour does not drain properly, pressure begins to build up (1). The optic cup is the most sensitive area (2), and the build-up of pressure can damage this cup (3), affecting vision. Glaucoma can result in a loss of sight at the sides (4).

behind the iris and surrounding the lens). After circulating through the pupil to the front of the iris, the fluid flows towards the trabeculum, which contains a structure called Schlemm's canal, through which fluid is absorbed into the bloodstream.

The pressure inside the eye depends on the amount of fluid in the eye, which depends on the condition of the drainage system. If the Schlemm's canal becomes blocked, the fluid

Shedding light on Van Gogh

The brilliant haloed paintings of Vincent Van Gogh are believed to be the result of glaucoma. In *Night Café*, painted in 1888, Van Gogh depicts three ceiling lights surrounded by yellow haloes. That is a common visual phenomenon with chronic open-angle glaucoma. Just after this painting was completed, the artist moved to the sunny south of France. That move may have been precipitated by the decreasing sensitivity that glaucoma sufferers have to light, and Van Gogh's resulting need to paint in brighter sunlight. It has been postulated that Van Gogh was not manic-depressive, but just depressed about his impending blindness.

level begins to build up, creating extra pressure. Because the weakest point in the eye is the optic nerve at the back, the pressure pushes the nerve into a concave or cupped shape. If the pressure remains too high for too long, parts of the optic nerve are damaged by atrophy (wasting away), and this results in a very gradual loss of vision.

The centre of our vision, where we see straight ahead or in reading, is not initially affected, but there is a loss of vision around the edges.

The most common form of the disease, open-angle glaucoma, affects about 250,000 Canadians. It progresses slowly as drainage in the trabeculum becomes increasingly blocked over time. With this form of the disease, the angle where the iris meets the cornea is open as wide as it should be. The entrance to the drainage canals can be seen with a special diagnostic lens and the canals should be working properly, but there is a clogging problem somewhere out of view. Imagine a sink with a partially blocked drain; the drainage of fluid becomes slower and slower, until water suddenly fills the sink. In the eye, the loss of vision begins very gradually, until there is noticeable deterioration in sight.

Why the drainage system clogs as we get older is not

known, but the problem is not life-threatening and seldom leads to blindness. It is not caused by too much reading, use of contact lenses, or any other function of normal living. Visual loss is both tragic and irreversible, but with proper life-long management the damage can be minimized.

Acute closed-angle (or narrow-angle) glaucoma is much less common. With this form, the drainage becomes blocked quickly and there is a sudden rise in pressure. This happens when the pupil dilates—going into a darkened movie house, perhaps, or because of certain eye drops. The iris bunches up over the drainage canals, plugging the outflow of aqueous fluid. This is more likely to happen if the angle between the iris and cornea is not as wide as it should be. People may have a genetic predisposition for this problem.

With closed-angle glaucoma, patients have severe headache, nausea, vomiting, eye pain, rainbows around lights, and blurred vision. This condition requires immediate attention. Treatment involves microsurgery or laser surgery (called iridectomy) to remove a small portion of the iris and open up the blocked drainage. This is usually very successful and long-lasting.

Secondary glaucoma can result from an eye injury, inflammation of the iris (iritis), an eye tumour, or advanced cataracts or diabetes. Treatment depends upon whether it is chronic or acute. Low-tension glaucoma, a very rare form, causes damage to the optic nerve despite the fact that the pressure is within normal limits. Why some optic nerves are hypersensitive and become damaged by normal eye pressure is not known.

Although glaucoma can occur at any age, it is far more common in those over the age of 35, and particularly among people with diabetes. There may be a tendency to inherit the problem, and it also seems to occur more frequently in the black population. A small percentage of infants suffer from what is known as congenital glaucoma. This can be an inherited condition, and results from incorrect or incomplete development of the child's eye's drainage system. Microsurgery must be used to correct these cases.

Internal eye pressure can be checked as part of a routine eye exam at any age, and thoroughly checked starting at age 35. After age 40 it should be measured every couple of years or, if there is a family history of the problem, every year. Measuring eye pressure is not a complete test itself, because pressure can vary depending upon the time of day and even the time of week. The sensitivity of the optic nerve can also vary, so that pressure that sometimes appears normal may still cause damage.

When glaucoma is suspected, five factors are checked:

- pressure within the eye
- shape and colour of the optic nerve
- colour vision
- the complete field of vision
- the filtration angle where the iris and cornea converge (the trabeculum and Schlemm's canal).

Tonometry measures the internal eye pressure and is the most crucial aspect of any screening for glaucoma. Anaesthetic drops are used to numb the eye and then a very small amount of pressure is applied by a tiny optical prism that is placed directly on the eyeball, or by a puff of air directed at the cornea. The doctor measures how much pressure is necessary to cause a slight indentation on the cornea. Normal pressure is 8 to 22 mmHg.

The hand-held ophthalmoscope (described in Chapter Two) is used to examine the back of the eye and the optic nerve. A nerve that is cupped in shape, or not a healthy pink colour, will be further evaluated by the ophthalmologist. If any other abnormalities or suspicious areas are detected, more tests will also be ordered. Next, a complete field-of-vision test is performed to attempt to locate any loss of sight at the periphery or outer limits of vision. All normal eyes have a small blind spot, but in glaucoma the blind spot (or scotoma) can become enlarged and can be mapped. If glaucoma is diagnosed, this test should be repeated once or twice a year to monitor changes and any further enlargement of the blind spot.

The simplest way to test the field of vision is to have the person cover one eye and stare straight ahead at the doctor's nose while the doctor moves a finger in from the side until the patient can first see it. This is done from the top, the sides, and the bottom, and is suitable as an initial screening test to find any gross deficits in the visual field.

A slightly more sophisticated and accurate test involves having the patient stare at a black screen with tiny white test objects moving into the middle. The patient tells the examiner when he first sees the test object, and the spot is marked so that a visual field can be plotted. If greater precision is required, a computerized test can be done using what is called a visual-field analyser, or octopus visual-field test.

The patient's head is positioned in an apparatus and the patient is told to stare at a fixed object that is straight ahead in the machine. A series of tiny lights are projected, and each time the patient sees a light he or she presses a button. The computer records which lights were seen and how intense they had to be before they could be seen, and a picture or graph of the visual field is printed out.

Gonioscopy is the process of examining the angle of the eye where the cornea meets the iris. An angulated mirror is mounted within a hand-held contact lens that is applied

Field of Vision

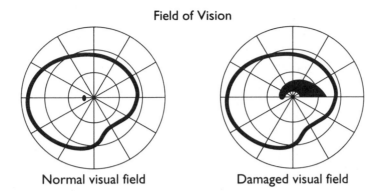

Normal visual field   Damaged visual field

The solid line indicates the extent to which an individual can see out the sides while looking straight ahead at the dot in the centre of the diagram. The black dot to the left of the centre is the normal blind spot. In glaucoma, the blind spot becomes enlarged, as is shown in the diagram on the right.

directly to the surface of the cornea. The doctor can then look into the mirror with the aid of the slit lamp, and see the iris and the anterior chamber angle magnified. This helps determine whether the patient has open-angle or closed-angle glaucoma and whether the condition is chronic or acute.

Treatment for chronic glaucoma begins with eye drops or oral medications to reduce pressure in the eye by decreasing production of the aqueous humour, or to open up the drainage spaces. Reduction in the aqueous humour is accomplished by two drugs called timolol maleate and betaxalol hydrochloride. They are part of a group of drugs called "beta-adrenergic blockers." These drugs may cause a slowing of the heart rate, lowered blood pressure, respiratory or cardiovascular distress, and possibly depression. They are not used on people with asthma. They do not affect the size of the pupil and so have little effect on vision.

Some drugs that improve drainage in the blocked trabecular channels must be used several times a day, every day, and they constrict the pupil. The oral medications acetazolamide, methazolamide, dichlorphenamine, and ethoxzolamide will also reduce the pressure, but they cause tingling in the extremities and a loss of appetite, and may be difficult for diabetics to tolerate. They also depress the potassium level in the blood and are known to cause kidney stones.

Over the course of your treatment, glaucoma medication may be changed or adjusted a number of times as the condition changes. This may not indicate that the glaucoma is progressing, but simply that your body is developing a tolerance to the drugs so that they are less effective. You may be able to go back to these medications after a year or two, when the tolerance wears off.

If eye drops and oral medications don't work, or you can't tolerate the drugs, surgery can be performed. The least invasive treatment is a procedure known as argon laser trabeculoplasty. After the administration of drops to anaesthetize the eye, the light beam is focused on a specific spot in the trabeculum and makes a microscopic burn. This opens the spaces and unclogs some of the drainage canals.

During the treatment, you will see a bright light similar to a camera flash and you may feel a slight tingling. Your eye may be slightly irritated afterward, but most patients require no further treatment. The operation can be carried out in the doctor's office or in an outpatient clinic, and the success rate is 80 to 90 percent. Usually only 25 to 33 percent of the trabecular area is treated at one time. Therefore, if the eye pressure remains high, at least two more argon laser treatments can be carried out.

In a few unsuccessful cases, microsurgery is necessary to

create an alternative drainage path. This is called a trabeculectomy. A space called a filtering bleb is created between the conjunctiva and the sclera to allow fluid to percolate out of the eye. In addition, a peripheral iridectomy is done, putting a small hole in the iris. The aqueous fluid formed in the ciliary body behind the iris now passes directly through this new hole in the iris, and on through the new trabeculotomy channel to the conjunctiva, where it is absorbed. This is an effective procedure with very few complications, although minor adjustments may have to be done after the initial surgery. Anti-inflammatory drops are used to prevent any scarring and to improve the outflow of fluids. A patch and an eye shield are usually worn for one day, and drops are used for about three weeks.

Acute glaucoma must be treated as an emergency to prevent damage to delicate eye tissues, primarily the optic nerve. First, drops are given to constrict the pupil and pull the iris away from the drainage system. Other drugs are used to lower the pressure. Then a small hole is made in the iris with the YAG laser. This procedure takes about 20 minutes, and the patient should remain in the office for a few hours after the laser treatment while the pressure is monitored. Success rates are high and complications are minimal. If the laser fails to lower the pressure, a surgical peripheral iridectomy is performed in the operating room; a small piece of the iris is removed to allow the eye fluid to drain properly even if the pupil dilates abnormally. This is usually a lifelong cure and eye drops are not normally required.

After microsurgery, patients are advised to keep water out of the eye, and to avoid driving and strenuous exercise for several weeks. In a few cases, the new drainage canal begins to close over and the pressure rises again. This happens because the body assumes the opening is an injury. Microsurgery can, if necessary, be repeated a few times in the same eye. Usually the laser is used to reopen a drainage channel that appears to be closing, and a second operation is avoided if possible.

It is important to tell any other doctors you may see that you are being treated for glaucoma, because some of the medications have side effects on other parts of your body, and treatment that you receive for other conditions may affect your glaucoma. If you are being treated by a cardiologist, dermatologist, or any other physician, make sure he or she is told about your eyes. Even if you take a common over-the-counter drug, check with the pharmacist about any effect it may have on your eye pressure. Some cough medicines, for example, can affect eye pressure.

Of course, you should watch carefully for changes in your vision. Any excessive irritation, watering, blurring, discharge, cloudy vision, headaches, flashes of light, floating objects in your field of vision, or haloes should be reported to your doctor. These could indicate anything from a simple eye infection to the need for a change in medication to a condition serious enough to require an operation.

Macular Degeneration

Jerry noticed one day that his right eye was slightly blurred. He closed that eye and he was able to see much more clearly with the left eye. As he hadn't been for an eye check for some time, he made an appointment with his ophthalmologist and described the problem.

Jerry was asked to look at a plate with vertical and horizontal lines about 3 mm apart. He noticed that the lines looked curved. The doctor then studied his retina very carefully and noted that there were changes in the macular area. These changes weren't very severe, but they had resulted in a decrease in vision from 20/20 to 20/40 in the right eye.

Jerry was given a copy of the line chart (called an Amsler Grid) to take home with him so that he could monitor his own vision over the next three months. About a month later he noticed that the distortion of the lines was getting worse, and he returned to his doctor. The degeneration of the macula was progressing.

Jerry was put on multivitamin zinc pills. Three months later his macular deterioration seemed to have stabilized. His vision, which had been 20/60 at the previous checkup, had remained the same.

But Jerry didn't bother to test himself regularly with the Amsler Grid, and at his next visit, four months later, his vision was down to 20/80. Within a year, his vision had deteriorated to 20/400 and he had no central sight remaining; he could see perfectly at the edges, but all he could see straight ahead was a black smudge. His other eye was now beginning to degenerate as well. At this point, he was referred to a Low Vision Centre at the local hospital, where various types of visual aids were available.

What is macular degeneration?

Macular degeneration is one of the most significant and frustrating causes of visual loss in the elderly. It causes a loss of central vision, as a result of either age-related deterioration of blood vessels or the abnormal growth of blood vessels in the macula—the most sensitive central portion of the retina, and the area that gives us our sharpest vision.

Involutional macular degeneration is the slow breakdown

of the structure of the macula, and accounts for about 80 percent of all cases. Exudative macular degeneration results in a very rapid loss of vision when abnormal new blood vessels leak or bleed into the macula.

At the moment the risk factors for this disease aren't clearly understood, but it appears that heredity, nutritional deficiencies, arteriosclerosis (hardening of the arteries), high blood pressure, smoking, and exposure to ultraviolet light may be implicated. As noted in the discussion of cataracts, all these problems are caused by or can increase free radical pathology. It has been suggested that anti-oxidant vitamins may help prevent macular degeneration, and that zinc may also help. Macular degeneration is more common among whites and those with light-coloured eyes.

The earliest symptom in both forms of macular degeneration is a gradual blurring of the central vision that interferes with activities such as reading and sewing. Often the condition is noticed on routine eye exams. The doctor may see tiny yellowish deposits or degenerative matter in the macular area of the retina, or the normal structure and pigmentation of the macula may be noticeably altered. Both eyes are usually deteriorating, although one is generally worse than the other. Many people are only minimally affected, and are able to compensate with better glasses and other visual aids such as reading glasses and halogen reading lights.

Amsler, a Swiss ophthalmologist, developed a series of lined and patterned grids for testing the central twenty degrees of the visual field. The subject covers one eye and looks at a central dot, and then describes any areas that appear distorted or interrupted. Both eyes can be tested and distortions can be documented for future comparison. People who have macular degeneration or who may be prone to it are often advised to keep a copy of this grid at home and to test themselves regularly.

Severe visual loss can occur in people with exudative degeneration caused by bleeding, fluid accumulation, and later scarring due to the presence of the tiny abnormal blood vessels. But even though the macula may be badly damaged, only central vision is lost. The remaining 95 percent of the retina is often unaffected. Some people with the exudative form are helped by laser therapy, if the problem is caught in time. A beam of laser light is focused on the retina to close the leaking blood vessels and to destroy the abnormal new ones. Lost vision cannot be restored, but the visual distortions may decrease and the progression of the disease may be halted. The problem often requires frequent monitoring, and perhaps further treatments with the laser.

S I X

Other Common Eye Problems

Blepharitis

There are two forms of blepharitis or inflamed eyelids—acute and chronic. Acute blepharitis is caused by a microorganism and is treated with antibiotic drops and ointment.

The chronic form can cause a type of eczema, with rough redness and flaking around the margins of the eyelids. There may also be an associated conjunctivitis with a loss of eyelashes. The first course of treatment should involve washing the eyes gently with warm diluted salt water two to three times per day. If that does not help, then the doctor will prescribe medication. A culture may have to be done to determine the exact cause of the condition. Allergy tests are also sometimes required.

> ## The History of Corneal Transplants
> The idea for corneal transplants was suggested as early as 1771, but the first corneal transplant wasn't performed until the early 1900s. A Moravian surgeon named Zirm transplanted the cornea from a young boy into the eye of a man who had been blinded by a lime splash. Today, with the vast array of instruments and steroids and antibiotics, the procedure is successful nine times out of ten.

Corneal Transplants

When it comes to organ transplants, people usually think of hearts and kidneys, but corneal transplants are the most common and successful of all the transplants done today. About 3 000 such transplants are done annually in Canada.

Traumatic injury such as a burn or penetration by a sharp object can permanently damage the cornea. Severe inflammation (called keratitis) from various bacterial or viral infections can also do permanent damage. In other cases, too much aqueous humour leaks into the cornea and it swells up so that vision is lost. There is also a rare disorder called keratoconus, in which the central corneal tissue thins and bulges forward, and permanent scarring can take place.

If your cornea is damaged beyond repair—and if you are healthy and you have no other major eye diseases—you will receive a cornea from a deceased human donor. The technique is called a penetrating keratoplasty, and it's done under a microscope. A round cookie-cutter type of instrument called a trephine is used to remove the central two-thirds of the damaged cornea. Next, a comparable piece of donor tissue is grafted on. The grafted tissue is sewn in place with nylon sutures that are finer than a strand of human hair. Antibiotics are given to reduce the risk of infection. The surgery takes 1 to 2 hours.

Total hospital stay is not usually more than a couple of days. Medicated drops are prescribed and you wear a patch at night and while washing to protect the eye. As with any transplant, rejection of the foreign tissue by your own immune system is a possibility. Redness of the eye, light sensitivity, and deteriorating vision may signal rejection, and the doctor should be consulted immediately. Prompt treatment can often reverse the rejection.

The transplant is normally clear within 2 weeks but full recovery can take up to a year. Astigmatism can be a problem but it may be alleviated by gradually removing the sutures, or contact lenses may be required. The success of transplants tends to be best in people with keratoconus, and much poorer for those with chemical burns from lye or acid.

Some ophthalmologists are now experimenting with the cool excimer laser (see Chapter Four) to smooth out scars in the cornea. This eliminates the need for corneal transplants in cases where the scar in the cornea is superficial, and it can be done very simply and quickly.

Corneal Ulcers

Corneal ulcers develop acutely as a discrete infected area invading the corneal tissue. The eye will be uncomfortable, even painful. The white of the eye may look reddish, and the ulcer may be visible as a distinct small misty area. Ulcers can be caused by injuries or infections, especially cold-sore infections such as herpes. You should never touch your eyes after touching a cold sore. Regardless of the cause, a corneal ulcer needs immediate attention. Eyes have been lost and blindness caused from neglecting a corneal ulcer.

Detached Retina

Gail was walking along the street when she suddenly noticed a dark cloud descending over her vision. She rubbed her eyes, thinking something had been blown into them, but the cloud remained. It covered about a third of her upper vision. Gail called her eye doctor and was told to come in immediately. She was diagnosed with a retinal detachment, was admitted to hospital, and had an operation that same day. Because of her immediate call to the doctor, almost all of Gail's vision was restored.

What happened to Gail was that the retina of her eye became separated from the outer layer. This can affect small areas or large sections, and can result in blindness if it is not treated very quickly. A hole or tear develops in the retina, and the eye fluid passes through the hole and separates the retina from the adjacent tissue.

Detached Retina

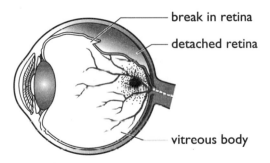

With a detached retina, the retina pulls away from the edge of the eye and develops a hole.

Injury to the head or the eye can also cause the problem. The vitreous body may begin to pull on the retina, making it detach. Inflammation and scarring can lead to detachment as well, but most cases stem from holes or tears.

A condition called "lattice degeneration" of the retina, often seen in patients with myopia, makes a person more susceptible to retinal detachment. In this condition the outer edges of the retina start to degenerate and therefore become very susceptible to developing holes. Shortsighted people should have regular retinal evaluations after the age of 40; small retinal holes can be treated by laser.

"Flashes" and "floaters" in the vision can be a sign that the retina has become detached, although they are usually seen with an otherwise normal retina. The sudden awareness of bright flashing spots and dark moving specks in front of the eye, with a black cloud coming over the visual field, is the first sign of a problem. The flashes are caused by the pull of the vitreous body on the retina, while the dark spots are caused by blood specks and vitreous condensations. But these signs can also result from a minor change in the vitreous body called "vitreous detachment," and only an ophthalmologist can distinguish between the two.

Retinal detachment may go unnoticed for a long period, until a substantial section of the retina has become detached. Suddenly the person will notice that a large section of vision is missing. The sensation is often described as a curtain or veil covering part of the visual field.

Before modern surgical techniques, detached retinas usually led to blindness. Today, the success rate for surgery is about 95 percent. Nonetheless, fast action is required. The retina requires nourishment and oxygen from the underlying blood vessels, or its rod and cone cells will die quickly. If the macula becomes detached as well, the chance of full recovery is much poorer. Once the cells are dead, they can't be replaced.

If the retina is torn but not detached, the doctor may be able to prevent detachment with a laser treatment. The procedure is known as photocoagulation and is done in the doctor's office or at a hospital clinic. The eye is anaesthetized and a special mirrored contact lens is placed on it so that the retina can be seen in sharp focus. Small laser burns are then applied to the edge of the retinal tear, like welds. The scars seal the edge and prevent the vitreous body from leaking behind the retina.

Laser treatment for retinal problems is not normally painful. The vision may be blurred for a short period after treatment, but this clears and vision is as good as it was prior to the problem.

Freezing (cryoretinopexy) is another simple method for repairing tears, and can also be done in the office or clinic. Using an ophthalmoscope, the surgeon places a small frozen probe on the sclera above the tear. The freezing extends into the retinal tissue and causes inflammation. The purpose, as with the laser, is to seal the tear with scar tissue.

For larger tears or complete detachments, major surgery in hospital is required. A piece of silicone rubber or silicone sponge is sewn to the outside of the eye to force the underlying tissue towards the separated retina. A laser or frozen probe is then used to scar the edges and seal the tissue onto the retina. The doctor may first have to drain the fluid beneath the retina, to bring the separated retina closer to the adjacent tissue so the scar formation will be strong enough to keep the two layers attached.

In other cases, the vitreous body is removed completely (this is called a vitrectomy) and replaced with a clear vitreous solution or special gases that push the retina back onto the underlying tissue. The original vitreous body will not be replaced, but the eye will make its own replacement fluid and vision will not be affected. If the retina is still not in the proper position, an air or gas bubble is injected to flatten it out.

Previously, patients had to remain immobile for months after this surgery so that the retina would heal. Today they are often out of bed the next day, and home within a few days. If air or gas bubbles are used, immobility may be required for a few days. The success of the surgery may take months to determine, and further detachments may occur.

Diabetic Retinopathy

Diabetes mellitus can cause many problems with vision, including:

- fluctuations of myopia (nearsightedness)
- eye muscle weakness and paralysis
- retinopathy.

Diabetes is a condition in which the body is unable to regulate its blood-sugar level. Diabetics take insulin to balance their blood sugar, but fluctuations still occur. When the blood sugar becomes elevated, there may be an increase in nearsightedness, because the lens of the eye swells. The diminished vision can be treated by stabilizing the blood-sugar level.

Eye muscle problems can also occur, resulting in the sudden development of double vision. This problem usually clears up on its own. Diabetes results in the paralysis of

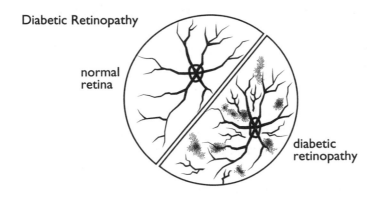

The retina on the right, that of a person with diabetes, has numerous abnormal blood vessels in it that break easily and bleed. The normal retina at left is shown for contrast.

peripheral nerves (called peripheral neuritis) and the ocular muscles are the most affected by this.

Diabetic retinopathy is a much more serious condition. It may not cause vision changes at first, but must be watched for carefully. The probability of a person with diabetes developing this problem increases with time, and reaches 75 percent after 20 years with the disease. It is one of the leading causes of blindness among diabetics over the age of sixty-five.

In one form of the condition, background retinopathy, some blood vessels shrink while others become enlarged and start to leak. Blood seeps into the retina, causing it to swell, and this eventually decreases vision.

In the more serious form of the condition, proliferative retinopathy, some of the blood vessels actually shut down, cutting off the nourishment to the retina. To make up for this, the retina begins to produce new blood vessels, but these new vessels are weak and fragile. As a result, they are more liable to burst and bleed into the vitreous body and the retina.

The leaking blood vessels of background retinopathy can be treated with the laser. A fluorescein angiogram is done to identify the leaking vessels. This test provides a detailed examination of the blood vessels of the retina and surrounding tissue at the back of the eye. Fluorescein dye is injected into a vein in the arm and circulates throughout the blood vessels, including those in the eye. A special camera takes high-contrast pictures as the dye flows through the retinal arteries and the veins of the inside of the eye, and blood leakage, macular degeneration, and blood vessel clots are identified. The laser is then used to seal off the leaks. If bleeding is more generalized, the laser will be aimed at the entire area involved, or a large portion of it, to seal off as many blood vessels as possible. This treatment may restore vision and prevent further deterioration, but it will not stop any new leaks from beginning, so it may have to be repeated a number of times.

In the case of the serious form, proliferative retinopathy, a method called panretinal laser photocoagulation is used to destroy the dead areas of the retina and prevent new, weak vessels from growing. Vision loss can't be reversed, but at least the progression will be slowed. The patient may experience some loss of side or night vision. Blurring is also a common side effect, but that often clears up.

If too much blood seeps into the vitreous body, laser surgery will not help and the physician must perform a vitrectomy. The vitreous body is broken up and suctioned out, and the cavity is filled with a replacement solution so the eye will retain its shape. (This is identical to the procedure used in treating detached retinas.) This operation can improve the vision of some patients, but there are many potential complications such as bleeding and infection. There is also a slight risk of retinal detachment after vitreous surgery.

Entropion and Ectropion

Two minor but irritating problems that are particularly likely to occur in older people are entropion and ectropion.

In entropion, the eyelid turns inward so that the eyelashes rub against the cornea. This results in the constant sensation of something being in the eye. If the condition is not corrected, there may be permanent damage to the cornea. Treatment consists of coagulating the base of the offending eyelashes with a very fine coagulating needle, similar to the type used to remove unwanted facial hairs.

In ectropion, the opposite happens—the lower eyelid hangs loose, turning outward. The tears from the lacrimal gland cannot reach the junction of the lacrimal canal in the inner corner of the lower eyelid. As a result, the tears continually run down the cheek. This problem can be corrected by minor surgery.

Exophthalmos

When tissue swells or builds up behind the eyeballs, pushing them forward in their sockets, the eyes may appear to be bulging. An abnormal amount of the white of the eyes may be visible, giving a "staring" effect. This condition is called exophthalmos, and it can be caused by a number of different disorders, but primarily by a thyroid condition. An ophthalmologist should be consulted.

Lumps around the eyes

If you develop a painless swelling on your eyelid, it may be a chalazion (also called a meibomian cyst). Chalazions are caused by blocked glands around the base of the eyelashes. They often go away without treatment but, if they persist, they can be easily removed by an ophthalmic surgeon under local anaesthetic. If a chalazion remains untreated and sore, see your doctor immediately.

Another form of growth is a papilloma or a growth of skin on the eyelid. Papillomas are harmless, but if they are unsightly they can be removed under local anaesthetic.

Yellowish patches sometimes appear on the skin around the inside corners of the eyes. These are called xanthelasma. They are harmless in themselves but their cause should be investigated. There may be an associated cholesterol problem involved.

Optic Neuritis

An inflammation of the optic nerve (optic neuritis) can cause blurred vision, eye pain, and even temporary blindness. The condition usually occurs in people between the age of twenty and forty, and generally goes away by itself. Even so, it should always be reported to an ophthalmologist. If it happens a second time, it could cause more serious damage. Optic neuritis accompanied by tingling fingers or difficulty in urinating may be a sign of multiple sclerosis.

Ptosis

If the nerve or muscle of the upper eyelid is weakened, the eyelid may droop, giving the eye a "sleepy" look and possibly obstructing vision. The condition, called ptosis, may result from accident or disease, or may develop in old age. Its causes should be investigated.

Ptosis can also appear at birth, as a result of an inherited tendency. Surgery by an ophthalmologist produces an excellent result.

SEVEN

Eye Emergencies

First aid for eye emergencies is limited by the fact that self-treatment may cause even more damage. A few basic first-aid principles are explained below, but the main rule to remember is that someone with a diseased or injured eye should be seen by a physician as soon as possible. Most hospital emergency rooms have full ophthalmic equipment, as well as an eye specialist on call twenty-four hours a day.

If someone has suffered a *blow to the eye*, manipulation of the lids or eyes should be avoided, and no ice or other substances should be applied. Eye patches are also not advised, as the pressure may aggravate any internal injury. Glasses, sunglasses, or a plastic eye shield may be used if they can be put on without any pressure to the swollen eye. The injured person should be taken to an emergency facility as fast as possible, by someone who can tell the doctor the time and circumstances of the injury.

The problems that can result from a blow to the eye range from simple swelling and bruising of the lid to haemorrhages, paralysis of the pupil, secondary glaucoma, fractures of the bone of the orbit, injured optic nerve, and detachment of the retina.

Danger Signals

When something goes wrong with the eye, it's possible for permanent damage to occur in a short time. If you have any of the following seven conditions, seek immediate medical attention, either from an ophthalmologist or at an emergency facility with proper eye equipment.

- sudden loss of vision or sudden blurred vision — this may be partial and may occur in one or both eyes
- sudden double vision
- flashes and floaters — that is, the perception of flashing or sparkling lights, with or without specks in your vision
- sudden marked distortion of vision, so that objects appear stretched or twisted
- severe redness of one or both eyes, with or without discharge, pain, or visual symptoms
- severe pain in one or both eyes, whether it begins suddenly or comes on gradually with or without nausea and vomiting
- any non-trivial eye injury, such as an eyelash or dirt in the eye, or a slipped contact that you can't easily retrieve.

If someone has had a *sharp injury to the eye*, first aid should only involve cleaning and dressing cuts and scrapes of the lids as much as is necessary to stop bleeding and prevent infection. If the lid is lacerated, it is possible that the wound extends into the eye, and a plastic shield or rigid protector, if available from a drugstore, should be applied very carefully. The person should try not to move the eye around, as this may do more damage. The object that caused the wound should be taken to the emergency facility for examination by the ophthalmologist. *If the object is embedded in the eye, it should be left there, as attempts to remove it may cause further injury.* In this case, transport the person very carefully—by ambulance if possible—to avoid moving the embedded object and doing more damage.

Foreign-body injuries are very common and not normally serious. Most foreign objects—like bits of grit, or fragments of hair—either sit on the cornea or become lodged under the lid, and can be well tolerated by the eye for a short time. Rapid blinking or holding the top lid over the bottom lid will stimulate tearing and wash the particle out, or the eye can be flushed with clean lukewarm water. No attempt should be made to remove particles with a cotton-tipped applicator, finger, or other probe, as considerable damage can be done.

If the irritation continues after the particle is removed, it may mean that the cornea is scratched. In that case, a doctor should be consulted immediately.

If blinking and tearing do not wash out the foreign particle, it may be so embedded in the cornea that it can be removed only with the aid of a slit lamp. In this case, an ophthalmologist should be consulted.

Any *dry or liquid chemicals* that touch the eye should be flushed out immediately with copious amounts of water. Most professional locations using such chemicals have special eye-irrigating stations, and if you work in such a location you should learn to—literally—find the eye station with your eyes closed. Any tap or water fountain can be used to flood the eye to dilute and remove the chemical. *Do not rub the eye*, and be careful not to flush the chemicals from an injured eye into an uninjured one. Once the eye has been thoroughly rinsed, the person should be taken to the emergency department immediately. Doctors there will need to know what chemical was involved.

If the eyes are exposed to extended or *severe glare*, such as direct or reflected sunlight or the flash from a welding torch, redness and discomfort may develop some time after the exposure. The eyes can be bathed with cool water and lightly covered with pads of clean, non-fluffy material. Then medical attention should be sought.

If you have overworn your contacts or fallen asleep while wearing semi-rigid gas-permeable lenses, you can cause corneal abrasions (scratches). If this happens and your eyes are red and irritated, and it feels like something is in your eye, see your ophthalmologist or go to the emergency room immediately. In addition to the usual eye exam with the slit lamp, fluorescein drops will be put in to better examine the cornea. If your cornea is scratched, you may need to wear a patch over the eye for a short period of time, as well as apply some antibiotic drops. You should only continue wearing your contacts after your eye has completely healed and with the approval of your physician.

On occasion, you may have difficulty removing a lens. If you cannot easily remove it, see your doctor or go to the emergency room as your attempts to find the lens may result in a scratched cornea or more serious damage.

Earlier in the book, we talked about the use of racquetball goggles and other protective devices after corneal and cataract surgery to prevent injury. Even if you have not had any surgery, have no problems with your eyes, and don't even wear glasses or contacts, it is essential that you use racquetball goggles for sporting activities. In fact, use of these goggles should not be restricted to sporting events. Woodworking and similar pursuits can also be dangerous to the eyes. A split second can result in serious damage to your eyes.

EIGHT

Environmental Modifications for the Visually Impaired

It is now possible for the visually handicapped to lead fairly normal lives. Society is, in fact, committed to improving the quality of life for people with all kinds of handicaps, and laws exist in many jurisdictions to make public buildings and areas accessible. But it's sometimes hard for the non-handicapped to appreciate the problems that have to be overcome.

What the visually handicapped need most are indicators and aids to help them orient themselves and move about safely. These range from simple devices like contrasting colours and embedded warning strips, to space-age electronic and biomedical sensory devices.

Home Modifications

A number of simple steps can be taken in homes in order to make life easier for those with low vision. If there are stairs leading up to the front door, railings should be installed on both sides. The railings should be painted in a bright colour which is different from the stairs. Stairs should be in good repair, with no loose flaps or uneven slats. Cocoa mats should be used in winter to reduce ice build-up.

The doorbell should be lit and the lock should be of a type that is easily opened with a key. Avoid scatter rugs in the foyer or entrance hall. Area rugs throughout the house are dangerous and wall-to-wall broadloom should be installed instead. All extension wires on the floor should be removed or nailed to the baseboards. No objects should be left that are less than about 60 cm in height. This would include such items as footstools and magazine racks.

If possible, use light switches that have a light on them. If that can't be done easily, then the light switch plate should be painted in a bright colour that contrasts with the colour of the wall. In the kitchen, cupboard door handles should be large and easy to grasp with the entire hand rather than with fingers. This would be of benefit to those who also have arthritis. Again, the handles should be brightly painted in a different colour from the cupboard door. Linoleum is the best type of flooring, as it is not slippery.

In the bathroom, both the tub and the toilet should be supplied with grab bars. Strips of adhesive should be placed in the tub to reduce the chance of slipping. The floor in the bathroom should also be composed of a granular surface, as soap and steam can make other types of floor covering very slippery.

Bright lighting should also be used everywhere in the house. If the stairs are wood, they should be covered with wall-to-wall carpeting to prevent slipping.

Public Areas

Many design changes are being made in public and commercial areas to make life easier for the handicapped and for those with low vision.

Doors should provide a clear opening of at least 80 cm, and doors designed for two people or one person and a dog should be at least 120 cm wide. Glass doors and other expanses of glass should have some marking to identify them, such as a colour decal that contrasts with the frame. Even people with normal vision bump into glass doors thinking that they are openings, so the decals, which should be at chest level, benefit everyone. The doorframe should be in a colour that contrasts with the wall surrounding it, and a contrasting floor colour also helps pinpoint the door.

Automatic doors should have guardrails, power floormats, a push or kick plate, and if possible an electric eye to keep them fully open until the person passes through. Revolving doors should have conventional doors next to them, and the colour of the doorknob should contrast with the colour around it. In addition, thresholds should be flush to the floor, and colour-cued. Floormats on either side of swinging or automatic doors should extend for the full swing area of the door as a warning of the area the door will cover.

Tactile floor signals and warning systems (such as raised or patterned areas) should be used wherever there are hazards to be avoided. These should provide a change in texture or hardness to alert the person that a hazard exists, and should be positioned well in advance of the hazard area—perhaps three metres ahead.

If a change in texture is used as the warning, that change must be distinctive enough to be detected by a cane. Glossy materials and those that produce a very bright reflection should be avoided.

Tactile warning signals should be properly placed to indicate stairways in the middle of a walk or corridor. Signals should also indicate the floor level. Improperly placed tactile indicators can cause tripping, so narrow grooves are preferable.

Those with impaired vision require more light than other people, but glare and reflections should be eliminated by using heavy matte surfaces, since low vision can make people very light-sensitive. Lighting should be used to accentuate stairs, handrails, decision-making points (intersections), restroom fixtures, and so on. Blinking lights should be avoided and very bright lighting should be provided in areas like stairwells.

Handrails should be placed on both sides of the stairs and should extend for an extra 30 cm at both the top and the bottom. The rails should be at least 70 cm inches above the stair and the endings should turn inward or downward to avoid dangerous projections. The colour of the handrail should contrast with the wall behind it.

Adequate lighting should be installed in elevators. Emergency control buttons should be grouped at the bottom of the panel, and should differ in shape, colour, and size from the regular buttons. The door casings on each floor should have the floor numbers marked by a raised numeral placed about a metre above the floor. Of course, talking elevators are preferable.

Routes to emergency exits must be well marked with tactile and audible warning systems. Doors to hazardous areas must be kept locked and audible warning signals on emergency doors should be standardized.

Restrooms should be located near entrances and main public spaces. Grab bars and toilet-paper dispensers should be the only objects surrounding the toilets. Adequate lighting should be provided and the faucet taps should have raised letters along with the standard colours for temperature. Signs on doors should be easily discernible by those with low vision; they should be at least 20 cm high, and the colour should contrast sharply with the door.

Large hazardous objects should be removed from all hallways, if possible, or at least be easily detected by a cane. Necessary protrusions like fire equipment and water fountains should be recessed. Furniture and other free-standing objects should be in contrasting colours. The underside of stairs and escalators should be enclosed.

For the benefit of people with reduced peripheral vision, signs should not be located where glare from the direct sun, low lighting, or shadows reduce visibility.

Room-identification signs and numbers should be raised, and information stations positioned just inside front doors should provide information for the visually impaired. This should include raised line-maps, personal assistance in orientation, and information about the building's signs. If the information is behind glass, non-glare glass should be used.

Alarm systems should be both audible and visual. The audible alarm should have an intensity and frequency that will attract the attention of people with partial hearing loss as well as visual problems.

External Areas

Entrances to buildings should be well lit and should lead into the main lobby. Entrances should have a faint tone or buzzer to assist the visually impaired to locate them easily, but these signals should be very faint so as not to confuse sighted people. Automatic door activators should be easily identifiable. Stairs and ramps should be clear of snow, ice, leaves, and litter.

Walkways should be designed to allow free access to buildings and adjacent streets. Hazards such as loose surfaces (gravel and stones) should be eliminated. Textural cues in the pavement should be positioned along the edges, and wide strips should be used so that they cannot be missed. Walks should not have gratings, since they are a hazard for canes. Overhead lights should be well out of the line of pedestrian traffic.

Ramps should be provided at crossings from walk to street level. Where intersections between walks and crossings are flush, tactile warning signals should be used and clearly marked. These signals should extend along the entire boundary between the walk and the street. Either paint or normal grey granite leading to a black asphalt road provides natural contrast. Crosswalk lines should be painted at all intersections.

Islands should comply with the same rules as sidewalks. Curbs should be raised to delineate islands clearly from the street. Like interior corridors, outside walkways should be free of hazardous objects: benches should not protrude into the path, and outdoor furniture, drinking fountains, phones, etc. should be well marked in contrasting colours and should have tactile warning systems.

NINE

Aids for Low Vision, and the Shape of the Future

The most significant advancement in the quality of life for the blind was the development of Braille. It was invented in Paris in 1829 by Louis Braille, who had lost his sight at the age of three. He had become frustrated with the bulky raised alphabet that was used to teach the blind to read and write. Braille spent a number of years developing a tactile code based on the placement of six raised dots.

For a number of years now, people with low vision have had large-print books and various types of magnifiers to enable them to read. With the huge explosion of technology in the past few years, the advancements being made to assist the blind and the visually impaired are as significant as the development of Braille.

Talking watches and talking calculators are not only available but reasonably inexpensive. A monocular (telescopic device) a little bigger than a jeweller's loupe can be carried in a pocket or purse and used to read house numbers or to check the number of an approaching bus. A portable lighted magnifier that magnifies ten times can also be carried about in pocket or purse and used to read. Even counting money is no longer a problem, as bills have (or soon will have) bar codes on them so that they can be scanned by a small optical reader.

A number of higher-tech devices for reading are now available, but the cost is still high enough to prevent most people from purchasing them for home use. They are normally found in libraries or offices. For example, books and papers can be placed on a platform where a miniature video camera photographs them and transmits the enlarged pages to a screen above. Cameras a little larger than a computer mouse can be used to scan a page of printed document and transmit the image to a monitor or computer screen. In addition, numerous computer software products will enlarge the print on the monitor according to the definition of the user. For example, for someone with only central vision, the image can be modified so that the cursor remains in the middle of the monitor and the text moves off to the left.

For people whose vision is completely gone, voice synthesizers will call out what is being typed or what appears on the screen. Software packages to do this require a separate keypad, and presently the quality of the voice makes it difficult to comprehend at first. People who are both deaf and blind, or who just can't get used to the voice, can use a Braille pad instead—this is a strip that translates what is on the screen into Braille. (Standard Braille uses six dots, but computer Braille uses eight dots; the extra dots indicate such things as capitals.) The controls to move the cursor around the screen are also in Braille.

The most remarkable piece of equipment is the "book reader," of which there are a few models. A book, newspaper, or document can be placed in the scanner and scanned within a few seconds; then it is read out loud. You can have the page read in its entirety, or request a paragraph, a sentence, or a word at a time. The speed can be varied, and you can choose voices from "frail Fred to beautiful Betty"; the quality of the voices is completely realistic.

Information about all of this equipment is available from your local association for the blind.

A recent development for people with very low vision is the Low Vision Enhancement System (LVES), designed by the Wilmer Eye Institute in Baltimore and NASA. It is intended for people whose better eye has vision ranging from 20/100 to 20/800—that is, people who can only see at 20 feet (6 metres) what someone with normal vision could see at 100 to 800 feet (30 to 240 metres). The device, which is worn over the eyes, consists of a miniature video camera, and two display monitors, less than two cm wide, mounted over the ears. The camera picks up objects and sends images to the monitors. Small mirrors reflect them from the screen to the eyes through prescription lenses. The LVES can focus from any distance to allow normal movement, zoom in for closeups of faces and reading material, enhance contrast, and display any type of video signal from a television, VCR, or computer screen.

The LVES weighs less than half a kilogram and is expected to cost about $3,000 U.S. To keep the cost down, only black-and-white is used at present, but eventually a colour model will be available as well.

By the end of the century, we may well have artificial eyes

for the blind. These will be tiny video cameras, either mounted on glasses or implanted in the eye socket. They will transmit images to the brain via a tiny wiring harness plugged into the skull. They won't enable the blind to see clearly, but they will provide the ability to see shapes and outlines, so that people can get around without white canes or guide dogs. Technology has actually advanced to the point where the microelectronics to do this currently exist. The sensor in home video cameras is only a few millimetres square and could be put into a tiny camera.

Producing more precise nerve cell stimulation in the brain has also been made easier with the development of the microelectrode. In early experiments, electrodes of about 1 mm in diameter were used, but were found to be too large. These electrodes were still about 50 times larger than the individual nerve cell. When one of these electrodes was stimulated, patients described seeing a small flash of light, called a phosphene.

However, when several electrodes were stimulated simultaneously to try to create a visual pattern, the results were varied. Because the electrodes were so much larger than the nerve cells, they tended to stimulate too many other adjacent nerve cells. The new microelectrodes are much smaller and closer in size to the actual nerve cell. Their tips can be placed closer to the cell so that they will require less current. They will then not stimulate as many other adjacent cells. Animal studies with these electrodes have demonstrated that the flashes of light or phosphenes can be produced over long periods of time without damaging the brain.

Dr. Gerald Loeb of Queen's University in Kingston, Ontario, and a team of researchers from the National Institute of Health in the U.S., carried out studies with three sighted patients who were undergoing surgery for epilepsy. The patients volunteered to have their surgery prolonged long enough to allow Loeb to stimulate the visual cortex which was exposed during the procedure. The patients then reported on the phosphenes that they saw. "The results," Loeb said, "were encouraging and provided critical information regarding the ideal dimensions for such electrodes. However, much more detailed information is needed than can be provided in a few minutes of testing time in the operating room."

As a result, in 1993, Dr. Loeb began experimentation with blind volunteers. Dr. John Girvin, a neurosurgeon in London, Ontario, who has been involved with these types of studies over the past 20 years, performed the surgery in Kingston. An array of about 16 microelectrodes made of extremely fine iridium and gold wires were inserted into the visual cortex by hand, using microforceps. Local anaesthesia only was used, so that the patient could tell the researchers if stimulation was producing phosphenes, thus indicating that the electrode placement was correct.

Once the electrodes are properly inserted, the bone is wired back in place and the scalp sutured. Rather than having wires come through the scalp, a small electronic package and a connector, each about 0.6 cm thick by 2.5 cm in diameter, is left under the scalp. The electronic circuitry stimulates and monitors the electrodes. It is powered and controlled by radio waves emanating from a small external transmitter that is placed on the scalp over them. This type of control system is known as telemetry.

Loeb stimulates the electrodes in a number of different combinations and intensities. He hopes to be able to get an accurate description of what the subject is seeing when different combinations of stimuli are applied. Even with only

16 electrodes, they expect to produce and to record thousands of different stimulus patterns and get thousands of responses from the subject.

If Loeb gets encouraging results, he can then use computers to simulate the way in which a functional visual prosthesis might work. This will enable him to answer questions such as how many electrodes are required to be useful and how the miniature video camera that will collect the images should be mounted.

Other researchers at the National Institute of Health in Bethesda, Maryland, have implanted an array of 38 electrodes deep into the visual cortex of a volunteer. The woman, who had lost her sight as the result of glaucoma, was able to see spots of light ranging in size from a pinpoint to a nickel. These spots were in red, yellow and green.

Scientists were able to light up six electrodes in a row simultaneously and the woman reported that she could see the letter "I". A unit with 250 electrodes is being developed that is hoped will create images by using dots of light in a manner similar to the way pictures are created on scoreboards when different patterns of bulbs are lit up.

Research to develop an artificial retina which would use the same principles as that for the cochlear or hearing prosthesis is being carried out at Johns Hopkins University in Baltimore. This device would electrically stimulate the retina. Researchers were able to stimulate visual light perception in three of four volunteers who had severe visual loss due to retinitis pigmentosa. This is a progressive degenerative disorder of the retina, for which there is no treatment, and which results in the destruction of the photoreceptor layer of the retina.

The intent of the work is to develop an array of electrodes that could stimulate the retina, allowing the individual to see the pattern that was displayed. Dot matrix printers use a 5 x 7 array that enables them to represent all letters. Research over the next few years will concentrate on the best method for stimulating the retina and increasing the understanding of the interface between the electrodes and the biological tissue.

Another approach to the treatment of blindness is the possibility of transplanting retinal cells to halt and reverse the problems of retinal deterioration associated with macular degeneration. Retinal cells have already been transplanted into blinded rats and about 20 percent of the vision of these rats was restored. The new cells are sensitive to light and able to process visual information quickly, and they transmit information to the proper region of the brain.

In yet another project, rats suffering from inherited blindness, or blinded by exposure to constant light, have had the death of photoreceptors temporarily halted by the injection of growth factors.

If the process is successful with animals that more closely resemble humans, and if the therapeutic agents are not too toxic, it may be possible to use the same principle on people.

Sight has been a mystery to us since the beginning of the human race. It has been revered as a divine gift, and feared as an inexplicable power. Now, as we explore the wonders of the space age, we may finally come to understand what goes on within the orbits of our own eyes.

Glossary

Accommodation — the adjustment of the eye for seeing at different distances. The shape of the lens is changed by the action of the ciliary muscle.

AK or arcuate keratotomy — the surgical procedure used to correct astigmatism.

Amblyopia (lazy-eye syndrome) — the inability of the eye to see, even though it is otherwise normal.

Amsler's Grid — a chart with vertical and horizontal lines, used to test for macular degeneration.

Angiography — a diagnostic method for outlining the blood vessels in the eye by injecting a material that can be picked up by X-ray.

Anterior chamber — the area of the eye in front of the lens, filled with aqueous humour.

Anti-oxidant vitamins—vitamins that counteract free radicals (see below) and neutralize them. Vitamins A, C, E and beta carotene are anti-oxidants and can be found in many fruits and vegetables.

Aperture-opening — the pupil is the aperture that lets light enter the eye.

Aphakic — vision without an internal lens. Aphakic glasses are used by people whose natural lenses have been removed and not replaced.

Aqueous humour — a watery solution in the anterior and posterior chambers of the eye.

Astigmatism — a visual problem where light focuses obliquely, caused by an irregular cornea or lens.

Automated microlamellar keratotomy — surgical resecting of the cornea to correct myopia and hyperopia.

Cataracts — a degenerative disease in which the human lens becomes opaque or cloudy.

Chalazion — also known as meibomian cysts, these are blocked glands around the base of the eyelashes that cause lumps around the eye.

Choroid — tissue between the sclera and the retina that contains many blood vessels and nourishes the eye.

Ciliary body — the part of the eye containing the muscles that change the shape of the human lens.

Ciliary zonules — ligaments that hold the lens in the proper position.

Cone cells — cells in the retina that provide the ability to see in bright illumination.

Conjunctiva — a thin membrane over the eye and the inside of the lid that protects and lubricates.

Cornea — the clear membrane over the eye, which bends light so that it focuses on the retina.

Cryoretinopexy — a method for repairing tears in the retina. The surgeon places a small frozen probe just above the tear which extends into it, causes inflammation and seals the tear with scar tissue.

Dark adaptation — the ability of the retina and pupil to adjust to low levels of light.

Depth perception — the ability to judge how far away an object is. The brain perceives depth by comparing the slightly different images from the two eyes.

Detached retina — the separation of part or all of the retina from the underlying tissue.

Diabetic retinopathy — an abnormal condition of the eye's blood vessels, caused by high blood sugar in diabetics.

Diopter — a unit of measurement indicating the correction necessary in a lens in order to properly focus light on the retina. A negative number indicates the correction needed for myopia while a positive number indicates the correction needed for hyperopia.

Ectropion — a condition where the lower eyelid hangs loose and outward and the tears cannot reach the drainage canal.

Edema — swelling due to an accumulation of fluid in the eye, usually seen in the cornea or the macula.

Endothelial cells — cells that line the back of the cornea and are needed for corneal transparency.

Entropion — a condition where the eyelid turns inward, resulting in the eyelash rubbing against the cornea and irritating it.

Epikeratophakia — surgery that sculpts human-donor corneal tissue into a lens implant.

Exopthalmos — abnormal protrusion or bulging of the eyeball.

Extracapsular cataract surgery — a technique where the front capsule of the lens is opened and cataract is removed manually.

Field of vision — the area that can be seen without moving the eye.

Floaters — small particles or cells that move about in the vitreous body and appear in the field of vision.

Fluorescein angiogram — fluoroscein dye is injected into a vein in the arm, circulates throughout the body and can then be seen and photographed in the blood vessels of the retina. Blood leakage from diabetic retinopathy, macular degeneration, and blood clots can be visualized.

Focus — the point where rays of light converge after passing through a lens.

Fovea — the very centre of the macula, where the most distinct vision takes place.

Free radical — an oxygen molecule with an odd rather than an even number of electrons. The extra electron results in an imbalance leading to instability, violent reactivity, and destruction of normal cells in the body.

Galactosemia — a congenital disease, resulting from enzyme deficiency, which affects the eyes and other organs.

Glaucoma — a build-up of pressure in the eye that can lead to blindness. Chronic or open-angle glaucoma is a slowly developing condition while closed-angle glaucoma comes on suddenly.

Gonioscope — a magnifying instrument used with strong light and a contact lens in order to examine the angle of the anterior chamber of the eye.

Hyperopia (farsightedness) — the inability to see close objects clearly.

Intracapsular cataract surgery — a technique where the entire cataract is removed within its capsule.

Iris — the coloured part of the eye, which contains two sets of muscles that control the size of the pupil, the dilator and the constricter.

Keratectomy — *see* Photorefractive Keratectomy.

Keratomileusis — surgical resculpting of the cornea.

Keratotomy — *see* Radial Keratotomy.

Lacrimal gland — a gland that secretes tears, located in the upper outer angle of the orbit.

Laser trabeculoplasty — a laser treatment to relieve the pressure of glaucoma.

Lazy-eye syndrome — *see* Amblyopia.

Lens — the small crystalline object behind the pupil, which helps focus light rays on the retina.

Light adaptation — the ability of the eye to adjust to variations in the amount of light.

Macula — the centre part of the retina, which gives us central vision.

Macular degeneration — the loss of central vision due to the deterioration of blood vessels in the macular area of the retina.

Meibomian cyst — *see* Chalazion.

Myopia (nearsightedness) — the inability to see distant objects clearly.

Occipital lobe — the area of the brain where we actually perceive vision.

Occluder — a device to block vision in one eye during an eye exam.

Ophthalmologist — a medical doctor (MD) who has specialized in eye care and diseases and eye surgery.

Ophthalmoscope — a hand-held instrument used to examine the inside of the eye.

Opticians — technicians who fill prescriptions for glasses or contacts from ophthalmologists and optometrists. Opticians are not permitted to test vision or treat problems.

Optic neuritis — an inflammation of the optic nerve that can cause blurred vision and even temporary blindness. It may clear up on its own.

Optometrist — an eye care specialist. An optometrist will have a doctor of optometry (OD) degree and is licensed to diagnose, manage, and treat some eye conditions. He or she may perform vision tests, prescribe glasses and fit contacts.

Orbit — the eye socket; the bony cavity that holds the eye.

Orthokeratology — the application of a series of different contact lenses, over time, to change the shape of the cornea.

Papilloma — a growth of skin on the eyelid or edge of the eye that is usually harmless.

Phaco-emulsification — the breaking up of a cataract lens by ultrasound and the removal of the material by suction.

Photocoagulation — the intentional burning by laser of parts of the retina or choroid in order to destroy degenerative areas.

Photorefractive Keratectomy — the correction of myopia and astigmatism using the excimer or cool laser.

Posterior chamber — the space between the back of the iris and the front of the retina, filled with the vitreous humour.

Presbyopia — a decrease in the ability of the lens to accommodate, that begins after age forty and leads to the need for reading glasses.

PRK — *see* Photorefractive Keratectomy.

Ptosis — a droopy eyelid caused by a weakened nerve or muscle in the eye.

Pupil — the hole in the middle of the eye that regulates the amount of light that enters.

Radial Keratotomy — the surgical procedure whereby small slits are made in the cornea to flatten it and correct for myopia.

Refraction — the bending of light rays by the eye to focus an image precisely on the retina.

Refractive error — the inability of the eye to properly focus light, leading to myopia, hyperopia, or astigmatism.

Retina — the sensitive part at the back of the eye that converts light into electrical signals that are sent to the visual cortex in the brain so that we can see. It is analogus to the film in a camera.

RK — *see* Radial Keratotomy.

Rod cells — cells in the retina that provide the ability to see in low levels of illumination.

Schirmer test — a test to assess the dryness of the eyes by leaving a paper strip in place for five minutes.

Schlemm's Canal — a circular canal where the cornea and sclera join and through which the aqueous humour is eliminated after it has circulated the ciliary body.

Sclera — the white protective part of the eye.

Scotoma — an area of lost or reduced vision, detectable in a field-of-vision test.

Snellen Chart — the common eye chart of rows of letters used to test vision.

Strabismus — a condition where the two eyes are not properly aligned and do not see the same object. This condition can lead to amblyopia.

Trabeculoplasty — a laser procedure used to burn tiny openings in the blocked trabeculum.

Trabeculotomy — the surgical removal of part of the trabeculum to improve the flow of aqueous humour in glaucoma patients.

Trabeculum — a network of small pores located where the iris meets the cornea and leads to Schlemm's canal. The trabeculum allows the aqueous humour to exit the eye, thus maintaining normal pressure. When the trabeculum is blocked, pressure builds up (glaucoma) and damage and blindness can result.

Vitreous body — a jelly-like substance behind the lens of the eye, filling the posterior chamber.

Xanthelasma — yellowish patches on the skin around the inside corners of the eye. They are normally harmless, but may indicate a cholesterol problem.

YAG laser — a cold laser using yttrium/aluminum/garnet, commonly used in eye surgery following cataract surgery and glaucoma.

Zonules — *see* Ciliary zonules.

Index